I0660543

Kept from All Contagion

SUNY series, Studies in the Long Nineteenth Century

Pamela K. Gilbert, editor

Kept from All Contagion

Germ Theory, Disease, and the Dilemma of
Human Contact in Late-Nineteenth-Century Literature

Kari Nixon

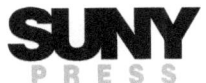

Published by State University of New York Press, Albany

© 2020 State University of New York

All rights reserved

No part of this book may be used or reproduced in any manner whatsoever
without written permission. No part of this book may be stored in a retrieval system
or transmitted in any form or by any means including electronic, electrostatic,
magnetic tape, mechanical, photocopying, recording, or otherwise without the prior
permission in writing of the publisher.

For information, contact State University of New York Press, Albany, NY
www.sunypress.edu

Library of Congress Cataloging-in-Publication Data

Names: Nixon, Kari, author.
Title: Kept from all contagion : germ theory, disease, and the dilemma of
    human contact in late nineteenth-century literature / Kari Nixon.
Description: Albany : State University of New York Press, [2020] | Series:
    SUNY series, studies in the long nineteenth century | Includes bibliographical
    references and index.
Identifiers: LCCN 2019027881 | ISBN 9781438478494 (hardcover : alk. paper) |
    ISBN 9781438478487 (pbk. : alk. paper) | ISBN 9781438478500 (ebook)
Subjects: LCSH: Communicable diseases in literature. | Germ theory of
    disease—History—19th century. | Literature and medicine—History—19th
    century. | Medicine in literature. | Literature, Modern—19th century.
Classification: LCC PN56.D56 N59 2020 | DDC 809/.933561—dc23
LC record available at https://lccn.loc.gov/2019027881

10 9 8 7 6 5 4 3 2 1

Contents

Illustrations

Acknowledgments

A version of chapter 1 was published in *Journal for Early Modern Cultural Studies* in Spring 2014. Likewise, a version of chapter 2 was published in *Journal for Medical Humanities* online in 2014 and in print in 2017.

Thank you to the Wellcome Library's online and physical holdings, and for their permission to use several images included in this book. I thank also Scholastic, for their generous permission to reprint a page from their magazine in this book.

I would like to acknowledge the support of SUNY Press as I went through the publication process, as well as Pamela Gilbert, the series editor. I am also grateful to the Sons of Norway for funding my research trips to Oslo to work on parts of this project, as well as the later funding of Whitworth University, which allowed my final trip to England in finishing this project.

I am forever grateful to the intellectual inspiration and guidance of my mentors, Ross Murfin, Beth Newman, and Rajani Sudan, who undertook the cultivation of a confused psych-school dropout and taught her the wonders of literary analysis and the medical humanities. I don't know that there will ever be words to fully express the impact you've had on my life in its deepest, intellectual understandings of the world—and because you all know me, you know that this speechlessness itself is rare. My loss for words of expression here is in fact the best indicator I can give of your profound influence on "this heart which beats / so wild, so deep in us—to know / whence our lives come and where they go."

No (hu)man is an island, as I will argue for the next several hundred pages, and I am no exception. The near-decade spent in penning this book also covered a decade of marriage, in which my unfailingly loving partner Daniel brainstormed ideas with me, read books alongside me, read over my chapters, waited outside of London museums while I conducted research, and stayed at home with an infant and a toddler while I went off to work to contemplate the past. Our late-night chats about my ideas, in which he traveled with me conceptually, have always been integral to my work. This book wouldn't exist without him.

To Betty and Mike: your support has always been more integral than you'll know. You never questioned my journey, and you've always been my cheerleaders.

For teaching me that we're all better off if we care about those around us—even when we might not be obligated to—I thank my parents, Anne and Kevin. The lessons about life and responsibility you taught me were undoubtedly foundational to the way I look at the world, history, and Victorian culture. Thank you also to my sister, Gracie, for teaching me the beauty of fearless love.

To Florence-Estelle (Flora) and Zelda-Elizabeth (Libby), I have only to quote Dickens:

> You have been in every line I have ever read. . . . You have been in every prospect I have ever seen since—on the river, on the sails of the ships, on the marshes, in the clouds, in the light, in the darkness, in the wind, in the woods, in the sea, in the streets. You have been the embodiment of every graceful fancy that my mind has ever become acquainted with. The stones of which the strongest London buildings are made, are not more real, or more impossible to be displaced by your hands, than your presence and influence have been to me, there and everywhere, and will be.

Your wondrous verve has taught me the revivifying value of human connection more than anything, at any price.

Introduction

"The Germ Theory Again":
Disease, Ideology, and the Possibilities of
Biotic Life in the World of Antibiotic Purity

Disease in the Community and the Self-at-Risk

In 1877, *Chambers's* magazine published an article wryly titled "The Germ Theory *Again*."[1] Although the article contains simply an uncontroversial historical summary of the concept, its very title belies the author's impatience with media saturation on the topic. Yet six years later in 1883, the London-based newspaper *Good Words* still found a demand for the topic, publishing a three-part series on germs titled "Microscopic Fungi" that eloquently reflects on the existential paradox of germs, those tiny "citadels of littleness" that wreak havoc on "person and estate."[2] The author empathizes with the presumed common attitude of his audience, agreeing "that it is hard to conceive how such immense capacity for evil gets stowed away in compass so small."[3] The tonal dissonance between these two publications highlights a key moment in history, in which I locate the goals of this project: the period between 1870 and 1900 when germ theory had "gone viral," so to speak—saturating media discourse and reaching a wide audience of popular science readers who engaged with and understood the concepts it embodied—and yet simultaneously remaining mystifying and rather terrifying to the audience that consumed knowledge of it so readily.

The growth, popularization, and prevalence of germ theory resituated the focus of scientific discourse on the humble microbe, and this conceptual priority in turn gave rise to the field of bacteriology at the end of the century. In a society just a decade beyond Darwin's famous publica-

1

tions, the synthesis of these cosmological and methodological frameworks underscored for Victorians an invisible battle waging all around them: the intricate interplay between microbe and mankind. By the 1870s (and after a half-century of seismic scientific paradigm shifts), the unending struggle between these two classes of lifeforms for superiority and survival—even as they often inhabit the same interstitial tissues and cells—was an ever-present reality for the reading Victorian public. Epistemologically founded on Darwinian concepts of survival of the fittest, methodologically bolstered by the microscopic findings of bacteriology, and conceptually familiar since the 1860s because of the widespread publication of theories of germs and contagion, human experience of the Anthropocene was resituated during this period. The human stage itself was now set, in the popular imagination, against a backdrop of other microscopic lifeforms hovering within, between, and amid the human bodies that had only recently seemed to predominate on earth. Thus, indeed, could magazines within the same ten-year period express both exasperation with germ theory as an overdone topic and also fearful wonder at the "unseen mist of organic atoms" and the "manifold evils they have wrought."[4] Certainly, this Darwinian struggle performed the destabilization of the Anthropocene—if not to the naked eye, then at least in printed narrative. Indeed, "Bulk has ever impressed [humans] powerfully . . . but these microscopic specks . . . had not bulk enough to startle him."[5] Here, the author expresses the common Victorian wonder at the terror invoked by tiny organisms, which had the power to resituate humankind as only one of a handful of powerful classes of being, rather than its predominant force. The author tracks the development of germ theory with succinct anthropomorphism, noting that humans, "till of late, knowing nothing of their mystery . . . had no dread of them. Now [they are] beginning to Awaken to truth, and with wider knowledge there has come a terror of small things."[6] This "terror of small things" must be seen, of course, as not merely a new and unexplored fear of the unseen, but a fear of a ubiquitous and omnipresent unseen. By the 1870s, nineteenth-century scientific cosmologies saw microbial life not as a series of invisible, separate particles, but an inescapable mass of potential contagion—a "mist" as this author calls it—that terrifyingly linked society together in a messy Petri dish of humanity, unheedful of social, class, gender, and sexual boundaries.

For many decades, in fact, this was the main and almost sole purview of germ theory—a new and unheard of realization of the interconnection of all human beings in a very physical sense that then led many Victorians (certainly not at a loss for overthinking) to consider the environmental, spiritual, social, and ethical networks of which they were inextricably a part. While Victorian awareness of social networks has been a topic of recent critical interest, such networks have thus far been theoretically and historically construed as seen rather positively by Victorians, revealing support and a common sense of welfare toward one another. But as germ theory and bacteriology would not bring about any practical medical cures until well into the twentieth century, Victorians, then, were situated at a very unique historical time in which they grappled with scientific findings that were almost purely conceptual. Certainly microbes could be seen, but what then? Cures were not emergent, and the public was left only with awareness of their universal risk via their very connection to the world and people around them. In this conceptual space, germ theory did very little *except* to highlight human interconnection in its most horrifying configuration.

Germ theory linked each illness to a specific microbe harbored in the human body and its waste, rejecting the older miasma theory's focus on unwholesome environments. Thus, germ theory moved the crosshairs of disease prevention from cleansing diseased *spaces* to cleansing or avoiding diseased *people*. What's more, the very nature of germ theory insisted on the actual, physical connection between bodies. The concept of social connection thus moved out of the realm of the theoretical signification into the realm of the hyperliteral—the very definition of the Kristevan abject. This in and of itself was enough to render germ theory horrifying to Victorians, for the overreal itself is horrifying. As Kristeva has illustrated, "in the presence of *signified* death—a flat encephalograph, for instance—I would understand, react, accept," but "the corpse . . . it upsets even more violently the one who confronts it as fragile and fallacious chance."[7] That this "hyperreal" connection, then, was by definition a connection of porous body to contagious porous body rendered the new conceptual stance nearly incommensurable with existence itself, since the human mind, as Kristeva has noted, "thrust[s] aside" these ideas "in order to live."[8] Bichat's early work representing interstitial tissue as an all-encompassing organ that delicately connects all of our seemingly disparate ones, effectively shaping them into the integral whole that we know as the body, could then be newly understood as but a microcosm for the whole of humanity.

Yet in this interstitially connected humanity the connective tissue itself was revealed as noxious, the abject that must be thrust aside (and yet never can be, for it is us) so that life as we know it to can continue, particularly when confronting "fragile and fallacious chance" in these risky encounters. Thus, while germ theory revealed the physicality of humanity's connections to itself and the world around it, it also simultaneously mutated this concept of connection into that which did not support the whole, but rather deeply threatened individual existence within the social body. That is, the social body could no longer be seen as a foundational critical mass upon which the individual body buoyed itself, but rather a cannibalistic force that threatened its own individual components by the very nature of its connectivity, now revealed as a palpable, physical (that is to say, no longer abstract) force. For Victorians, humanity itself seemed transformed into a cruel, inescapable murmuration in all its contagious and ubiquitous connectivity. Any preexisting notion of social interdependence, connectivity, and network culture was not merely underscored by germ theory, it was rendered literal, corporeal, and visible, if microscopic. Importantly, this connection ceased to connote notions of safety in numbers and supportive assistance and suddenly seemed to represent—in the same mass of people—hazard and risk. Benedict Anderson has argued that his famous notion of imagined communities was a concept "capable of being transplanted, with varying degrees . . . to a great variety of social terrains, to merge and be merged with a correspondingly wide variety of political and ideological constellations."[9] In this context, I will argue that community ideologically became an inescapable monster, and that this perception had real political and social consequences—often in the forms of Foucauldian surveillance and control that have become commonplace in Victorian studies, and largely for already marginalized populations. Community no longer signified aid through cooperative endeavors, but competitive organisms fighting each other for survival in a zero-sum battle against bacteria.

Various existential needs were at odds, then. To maintain a psychological sense of life in a world of risk, it suddenly seemed incumbent to avoid community (and risk) altogether in order to preserve bare, physical life (my debt to Agamben and his discussions of the way modernity places "biological life at the center of its calculations" should be here apparent).[10] As Kristeva says, in the face of "a flat encephalograph," we would give up—relinquish control of an obviously unchangeable fate. But confrontation with "fragile and fallacious chance" has the tendency to bring out human grit, as any and all apocalyptic films demonstrate. This perceived risk—not yet a death, not yet despair, but only an ever-present threat—and its biopolitical fallout in biological and existential life are what I aim to explore in this book, in the brief moment when Victorians grappled with these apparent realities freshly and in a completely unique conceptual space. Free from the complicating factor of practical solutions to these problems, Victorians inhabited a virtual thought experiment where these needs and values and their biopolitical implications can be isolated and explored.

Amid a scientific milieu that urged a fundamentally altered way of considering disease, then, I demonstrate that a set of late-nineteenth-century authors used the medium of fiction and drama to resist what they saw to be the troubling sociopolitical implications of these new epidemiological understandings. To this end, my project highlights the convergent chronology, but divergent ethical imperatives, of two parallel yet opposed narratives. Germ theory implicitly packaged into its rhetoric an advocacy of personal sanitation through meticulous disinfection and maintenance of asepsis via isolation from other potential disease vectors (i.e., other humans, in many cases), an increasingly authoritative approach. While this ideology often took the physical form of highlighting health and home sanitation, its work was often subtler, as images of isolation and risk aversion pervaded more and more literature of this period, and advertisements promoting products that guaranteed entire microbial sterilization became increasingly prevalent. This broad notion has been addressed in recent microhistories of germ theory, but I argue that we can glean a deeper cultural understanding of the bioethical impacts of such scientific frameworks by excavating the undercurrent of an opposed narrative built into the fiction of late Victorian authors who vehemently denied the positive *social* value of such attitudes and practices, even as its biological implications seemed clearly advantageous.[11] Instead, their fiction subverts germ theory specifically and unmitigated scientific authority more generally by defiantly and consistently illustrating intimate relationships as fruitful and meaningful in spite of—and sometimes *because of*—infectious contact. Moreover, many of these texts represent purity (microbial, moral, or otherwise) itself—that exemplar of what is often reductively used as a stand-in for "Victorian"—as exactly that: lifeless. The texts I cover here expose a shockingly modern depiction of purity as unpalatably sterile, devitalized spaces cleansed of life itself. Thus, the microcosmic and microscopic imperative of germ theory—to sanitize, scrub, and so fend off all contaminating influences—was deftly picked up by Victorian authors as a handy means of subverting the dominant paradigm of disease as a thinly veiled palimpsest for moral impurities. The authors who picked up on this means of protest are rarely connected in present-day literary criticism and come from a wide range of backgrounds and geographical areas. Yet, as they are so united in the causes I identify here, I have developed the term Biopolitical Resistance Literature to describe the joint aims of the work I cover in this period.

It is worth pausing in this epistemological history to note that in coining this phrase, I mean to develop a convenient way of describing works that engage in similar modes of rejecting a similar set of medically and scientifically informed ways of engaging in the world. While I certainly think the authors covered here *saw themselves* as resisting very particular behaviors that were informed by emerging science, it is worth clarifying the fact that I do not see these authors as self-aware themselves of a unity between their works or of a collective, identified agenda such as would have existed for New Woman Fiction, for instance. That is, in coining the term Biopolitical Resistance Literature, I aim to group like-minded authors together as a set in this book (and perhaps for other scholars in future work), who were all independently and conscientiously engaged in responding in very particular ways to very particular things. I do not intend to imply that the authors grouped under this term would have seen what they were doing as part of a collective movement at the time, but that these individual projects spontaneously responded to a similar set of criteria and thus wove several insistent, independent argumentative strains into a cultural tapestry of resistance to a set of late-nineteenth-century biopolitical norms. Nor can we assume that these authors would have used anything like a concept of biopolitics in understanding themselves, of course. I certainly will argue that they saw themselves as attacking norms of structuring community and the contemporary standards for ethics of human interaction. In my mind, these concepts, when structured and informed by public health initiatives and contemporary science, are most easily grouped under the element of biopolitics, but I wish to be clear in stating that this is our current term for understanding such dynamics; the Victorians would have seen this under concepts of community, engagement, and individual responsibility to a larger world.

To return to Victorians and germs, then, I argue in this book that by turning an age-old representational schema of purity and contamination on its head, authors of biopolitical resistance literature in this period pushed back against the problematic and literalized impacts of germ theory's tendency to catalyze isolationism, self-interested social Darwinism, and disregard for the common good. These authors saw this tendency for what it was and, realizing its problematic results for social justice and bioethics, turned the tools of this metonym against itself, constructing a countercultural narrative in which *pure* spaces and actions were revealed as not simply antiseptic and without contamination, but—as we now know antibiotic environments to be—incapable of sustaining thriving life. To find life-giving media (to use Petri's microbial term), we must take with it the risk that comes from other life forms. We must embrace our contaminated connectivity as the inextricably intertwined states that they are, and realize that to reject risk is to reject real connection with others.

Thus, in a world that had become increasingly invested in a search for new moral epistemologies after the findings of Darwin, Lyell, and others like them had chipped away at the authority of the church, authors of biopolitical resistance literature undermined convenient neoliberal ideologies of human value, and in this case held human community and social relationships as the highest good for mankind. Their fiction urges readers to avoid pitching neoliberal values of science as the newest Godhead, arbiter of behavior and purity, and instead to look to themselves and one another as mankind's only possible source of salvation. It may be messy, dirty, and even deadly, these authors suggest, but even potentially fatal interaction with the human community is ultimately more salvific than stagnant isolation unto oneself. There is some dissonance, then, between the few individuals that resisted the growing totalitarian claims of germ theory on modes of behavior, interaction, and purity, and the general cultural zeitgeist that was quickly gaining momentum in unquestioning support of this movement; it is this dissonance—a tension between cosmological polarities—that I explore with the following chapters. That there were those who resisted the claims of germ theory, and that such resistance worked against a general tide of unequivocal cultural acceptance, has been established in historical accounts. In the pages that follow, I aim to add epistemological depth to such accounts by exploring the cultural *effects* of such resistance. Although a fair amount of material is to be found about diseases specifically and sickness generally in the Victorian era, a broad literary history of germ theory grounded in explorations of its impact on the representation of different diseases and its implications for intimate interpersonal relationships has never been written yet, and such a history promises to be both revealing and fruitful.

All these existential reflections, of course, are possible because of the biophysical *realities* of the prevalence of infectious disease in the nineteenth century. As such, nineteenth-century fiction is likewise replete with disease, which became a vehicle through which authors could address the problems of selfhood and the self within a changing society. This vehicle was apt for the Victorians because of scientific developments in their century, but remains meaningful for us to consider today, because disease discourse is not purely scientific data about microbes multiplying or viral agents invading host cells. Disease matters to us because disease affects human bodies, rendering the sea of selves that constitute society suddenly nonfunctional, or at least less functional than modern normative parameters would like to allow for. Disease discourse is therefore replete with all the sorts of anxieties of independent selfhood and presumed-upon able-bodiedness that disability studies, queer theory, and gender studies have separately set out to critique.[12] My project aims to extend these critiques into the as-yet-unexplored realm of disease and illness. Just as Bruno Latour, Donna Haraway, Simon Schaffer and Steven Shapin, Roy Porter, and others have problematized Cartesian paradigms of universal, independent, natural agency, I argue here that the implications of disease discourse do not end with personal questions of identity maintained and protected in a medico-scientific vacuum—which the following authors vividly demonstrated. As Kristeva has shown, identity *cannot* be substantiated in a vacuum, but is founded first upon notions of who others are. The self in search of subjectivity must necessarily traverse definitions of others in the formation of a self that can only be conceptualized as a sort of negative afterimage. The self without society is itself *anti*biotic. Indeed, the very concept of probiotics was developed in the late Victorian era, presenting real relevance to their own sense that the literal and metaphoric were not distinct subjects in the discussion of life, macroscopic or otherwise. The Victorians were perceptively aware, more than a century before Kristeva and modern-day biopolitics, that what we talk about when we talk about disease is necessarily about the self, but is also just as necessarily about the others that surround the self. In the atmosphere of *contagious* disease, however, these subjectivity-producing boundaries of selfhood and otherness are destabilized. Perceived threat to these boundaries all depends, of course, on how one conceptualizes disease, and in the nineteenth century, this was not always so clear in the face of changing scientific epistemologies.

Building on recent historical analyses delineating contemporary resistance to germ theory's politically motivated "discovery," my project fleshes out the cultural ramifications of these reactions by considering a handful of novelists and dramatists who stubbornly reworked the hegemonic paradigm of purity as a universally recognized good, and instead depicted contagion nestled comfortably within community and camaraderie. These authors quite readily used contagion itself to underscore the importance of community interactions and the vitiating effects of isolationism. Rather than emphasizing aseptic isolation, the practical imperative of germ theory, these authors indicated instead that interaction in the messy amalgam of humanity was the only source of moral progress in an increasingly secular society. Authorial engagement with and understanding of contemporary scientific developments in the Victorian era is well known; germ theory was widely discussed in a broad range of periodicals, and most literate Victorians knew of contemporary developments in bacteriology. Voracious readers and publishers themselves, Victorian authors in particular often had their fingers closest to this *social* pulse of scientific data, building commentary about the import of such findings into otherwise typical Victorian plots. In light of this, my project argues that a great many late-century authors (often seemingly unrelated ones such as Thomas Hardy, Henrik Ibsen, and Mary Elizabeth Braddon) used their writing to depict the stifling world that a culture of "sanitary" isolation based on germ theory seemed to encourage. Rejecting germ theory's phenomenological implication that absolute purity is possible or desirable, these authors insistently portray the value of human connection, however contagious, and depict social connection as valuable and necessary in spite of (and often *because* of) contaminating disease, instead of portraying disease as evidence of failed sanitary preemptives.

Each of my chapters focuses on a particular disease—plague, streptococcus, tuberculosis, and syphilis. By focusing on individual maladies, I ground my argument in the specific social conditions surrounding each disease, making palpable the ethical imperatives of authors such as Ellen Wood and Ella Hepworth Dixon. Yet the range of diseases I address—pulmonary, venereal, bacterial—shows how writers' use of contagion broadly engaged the shifting conceptualizations of disease in this period. To make clear just how specific and incisive these authors' critiques were, I have moreover grouped each disease with a specific social or legislative concern with which it was discussed in tandem contemporarily, and which the authors at hand draw into their fictional discussions. Generally, each of these sets of diseases and their concomitant social concerns are portrayed in the fictional work through focused authorial attention on one type of human relationship; thus, each chapter is trifocal in nature: microbial, relational, and sociopolitical. By focusing on these three levels of human interaction, I am able to highlight the broad implications the ideological work of germ theory had. More importantly, however, I have chosen these parallel foci in each chapter, because they are the same structural levels I see the authors of biopolitical resistance literature using to make their claims.

By way of introduction, my first chapter looks back to Daniel Defoe's *A Journal of the Plague Year* (1722) and Mary Shelley's *The Last Man* (1826) to examine community strictures in times of epidemic, alongside authorial responses to them in a time well before germ theory began to show up as a term in public discourse in the 1840s. By highlighting texts that assessed widespread, apocalyptic contagion even before germ theory, I isolate and demonstrate the impact of disease discourse on society, especially when science-based legislation is at issue. In addition to looking more broadly at large community relations, I also address contemporary inoculation debates, which were increasingly common at this time.

For Defoe, isolation results in festering and further contamination. In *Journal of the Plague Year*, Defoe repeatedly depicts grotesque, noxious ruptures of contaminated material from sealed structures, bodies, and communities. Conversely, the successful characters and healthy spaces in the text are depicted via osmotic motifs that valorize bodies in continued circulation. Bodies—and for Defoe this includes bodies of trade, corporeal bodies, and international relations simultaneously—are effectively aired and ventilated through controlled flow within and between communities. In the cosmology he develops, this circulation is necessary for the vitality of personal, community, and national bodies. To a similar end, Shelley demonstrates the futility of successful isolation in *The Last Man* as she tracks her protagonists in their (largely) unsuccessful journey to isolate themselves from a London plague. Shelley employs topographical images of isolation such as island geography and mountain ranges to construct her view of isolationism as potentially protective, but generally more likely to result in the horrors of being cornered *with* disease and without resources, or, at best, being safe, alive, and utterly alone.

In discussion of both texts, I excavate authorial engagement with contemporary debates surrounding inoculation—the process of incorporating diseased matter into the body in a controlled manner in order to prevent being completely overcome by this same disease. This techne was promoted during the period of Defoe's novel, and increasingly urged in Shelley's time (in the form of Jenner's vaccination) as a universal mode of public health. Inoculation also sets the stage for my introduction of another term critical to this project as a whole—"risk encounters." Throughout the texts I highlight, I note authors promoting various forms of risk encounters that they in fact advocate as necessary for vitalizing individual and community progress. Both Defoe and Shelley, for instance, insist on this vitalizing importance of community, even though it was well known in the eighteenth century that plague, at least, was contagious. Their persistent communalism in the face of known contagious danger sets the stage for my broader consideration of the post–germ theory world, in which nearly *all* diseases, not just the bubonic plague, were understood to be communicated by the friends and family—the community—in which one lived.

After establishing the effects of epidemic on community mentalities—and authorial resistance to social isolationism by promoting risk encounters in their fiction—I turn to the post–germ theory era, when (as indicated by "Vegetable Villains" quoted above) microscopic findings seemed to reveal disease *everywhere,* lurking in every body with whom one interacted. My second chapter, "'A Speculative Idea': Childbed Fever, Early Germ Theory Debates, and (En)gendered Speculation in Henry James's *Washington Square*," explores the early development of germ theory in a transatlantic context using arguably the most British of American authors in the nineteenth century. By illustrating some of the early transatlantic debates regarding germ theory and the effects of this information upon a particular sociocommercial context, this chapter makes the first foray into elucidating the effects of germ theory upon popular culture and interpersonal relationships. *Washington Square* (1880) is in many ways a typically Jamesian novella—light on plot, heavy on character development, and seemingly anticlimactic in conclusion. Yet the novel's ending is radically different, I argue, if read in light of the contemporary debates about germ theory and their effect on the father-daughter relationship that makes up most of the novel. This chapter addresses one of the earliest novels I analyze from the late Victorian period, and importantly represents some of the earliest concerns surrounding germ theory. These concerns dealt largely with the potential for the newly emergent professional obstetrician to contaminate patients with a then-deadly strain of streptococcus. Because of its composition at a time when germ theory was widely and indeed feverishly accepted (the 1880s), and its fictional situation in a time before this was so (the 1830s), this novel is valuable as an initial illustration of the trajectory of germ theory's influence on late-Victorian culture. Moreover, James sketches out his female protagonist's reaction to the risk-averse culture of the androcentric medical profession that surrounds her and, I argue, ultimately resists an abiotic, risk-averse life.

Having sketched out the broad cultural impact of contagion as well as the history of germ theory's international development, my next chapters hone in on the Victorian era in Britain, exploring specific contagious illnesses and the social issues surrounding them during the advent of modern germ theory and bacteriology. Chapter 3 moves from the subject of familial relations to consider female homosociality; it compares metaphorical uses of tuberculosis as a vessel for representing the possibilities of female relationships with other women in female-authored texts that span the century, including Charlotte Brontë's *Jane Eyre* (1847), Ellen Wood's *East Lynne* (1860), Mary Elizabeth Braddon's *John Marchmont's Legacy* (1863), and Ella Hepworth Dixon's *The Story of a Modern Woman* (1894). Thus, this chapter straddles time periods in consideration of the changing and always slippery mythos surrounding disease using perhaps its slipperiest of nineteenth-century embodiments, tuberculosis. In this series of novels, each female protagonist withers away, literally stifled by her isolation from other women. In this set of novels, isolation does not purify, it putrefies, and exposure to risk is depicted as necessary and life-giving. By juxtaposing tubercular deaths across the century, this chapter explores the ways in which germ theory drastically changed not only the symbolic potential of this disease, but also how female authors repurposed this metaphorical energy to address social questions relevant to women. In doing so, I show that these female authors used their fiction to insist against the isolationist imperatives of germ theory—which they demonstrated to be often used to subjugate and harm women—and implicitly highlight the value of social encounters, however risky they may be.

Moving from homosocial relations to heterosexual intercourse, the fourth chapter deals with syphilis and sexuality in literature published and performed around the time of the repeal of the Contagious Disease Acts. This chapter works through juxtaposition, showing the ways in which conceptualization of disease changed not only in response to germ theory alone but also in response to political changes that were catalyzed by these changing scientific understandings of disease. In doing so, this discussion tackles intimate sexual relationships—both marital and otherwise—in the Victorian era. Chapter 4, "Tainted Love: Venereal Disease, Morality, and the Contagious Disease Acts in Ibsen's *Ghosts* and Hardy's *The Woodlanders* and *Jude the Obscure*," deals with syphilis and sexuality in literature published around the time of the repeal of the Contagious Disease Acts. In 1886, the Contagious Disease Acts were repealed. These laws—which attempted to control the spread of syphilis by allowing for the genital inspection of any woman suspected of being a prostitute (a stipulation that could apply to virtually any unescorted woman found out-of-doors after dark)—had been under attack for nearly two decades by burgeoning feminist organizations as well as periodicals such as *The Shield*, founded for the particular purpose of protesting the laws. Additionally, growing cultural awareness of the evidence of germ theory during this period—evidence that shed light on the specific microbiological agents involved in the spread of disease—was also of prime import in repealing the CDA. Women and doctors alike took to the political battlefronts with a veritable artillery of scientific evidence, arguing that women could not be solely responsible for the spread of venereal disease. Their efforts were aimed at protecting not only against forcibly "inspected" women, but also the misguided angels of collective society's houses who often innocently contracted syphilis from their husbands and passed it onto their children because of the misinformation surrounding the contagious nature of syphilis. Texts such as Sarah Grand's 1893 *The Heavenly Twins* famously take on this issue of women's sexual education.

However, this chapter seeks to call attention to the ways in which the changing understanding of epidemiology based on the new evidence of germ theory was also engaged by male authors seeking to upend the status quo through their fiction. To this end, this paper compares Thomas Hardy's 1887 novel *The Woodlanders* with Henrik Ibsen's play *Ghosts* (written in 1881 but first performed in England in 1891). Both of these works involve contagious sexual contact (fever contracted through oral contact and congenital syphilis, respectively) and both make striking statements about the implications of such contagion in terms of the standing social order. The representations of illness in both texts are complexly subversive insofar as they each intertwine contemporary medical and bioethical evidence into the tapestry of their stories, and urge readers to engage with risk encounters. In doing so, this chapter demonstrates even further the real political implications of disease conceptualization built into discussion of intimate sexual relationships, as well as returning to familial relationships in a discussion of the interactions of a mother and son.

In addition to opening Hardy's and Ibsen's texts up for more fruitful analyses of their progressive cultural work, reading these texts with an eye to germ theory evidence allows the close connections between the work of Hardy and Ibsen to emerge. Although one would be hard-pressed to deny their similarities in terms of tone and thematic purpose, virtually no scholarship exists that compares the two at length, and the striking fact that both men utilized the evidence of germ theory in works published within the same six-year period clearly indicates the utility of exploring the connections between these two authors in greater detail. The chapter concludes with an analysis of Little Father Time as a victim of congenital syphilis, a character who, in his diseased state, represents the haunting return of the repressed in this novel, the "nodal point" that undoes all the action of the plot. Thus, I complete this chapter by assessing a character that once again insists that self-protective isolation is neither fruitful nor possible. That is, Little Father Time's actions both morally castigate Victorian social norms which have led to his syphilitic condition (by mandating hidden sexual intercourses) and reject Jude and Sue's misguided attempts to simply eschew society altogether. Even in order to flout toxic social norms, Little Father Time's role seems to suggest, solutions *outside* of society—or, to put it another way, disregarding it—are untenable within the life of the social body.

Chapter 5 begins with this dilemma of attempting social progress outside of society. In Grant Allen's 1895 *The Woman Who Did*, the protagonist, like Jude and Sue before her, sets out to publicly flout Victorian sexual mores by living openly with her lover and by refusing to marry him on principle. However, her husband dies of typhoid fever during travel abroad, and the couple's daughter ends up resenting her mother's forced isolation of her from society and rebels by following the status quo to the letter. This letter, as Hardy notes in the epigraph to *Jude the Obscure*, "killeth." Indeed, Herminia is heartbroken when her plans backfire. She kills herself when her attempt at isolation—righteous though it may have been—end in her total loss of a relationship with her daughter. As mentioned earlier, her husband dies, having contracted his illness during the couple's attempt to physically move away from the space of British social norms by traveling to Italy. In this chapter, then, I cross-reference the previous concerns of the volume, which take up issues of women's social networks and isolationist tendencies in the wake of disease, and apply them to this novel, which features a woman who attempts to isolate herself from what she sees as the *diseased morality* of the available social networks—to no better end than her literary forebears. I connect this reading with another Ibsen play, the one he wrote immediately following *Ghosts* and which, I argue, further develops his notions on the subject. Both *The Woman Who Did* and *An Enemy of the People* incorporate typhoid fever into their work, drawing upon cutting-edge ideas of probiotic sewage breakdown to insist on openness and connection, even when taking on the establishment.

Building from Herminia's failed social experiment, I then present a revisionist reading of Ibsen's *An Enemy of the People*. I view Dr. Stockmann not as he is generally viewed (as an environmental and social advocate dedicated to cleansing the town of cholera), but as a character through whom Ibsen denounces both unmitigated authority and unregenerative purity, moral and microbial. When Dr. Stockmann is run out of the town hall with cries of "Folkefiende! Folkefiende!" echoing behind him, he is traditionally read as a man of high moral aims victimized by the middle-class masses jealously protecting their profit and power even though lives are at risk. Yet Stockmann, who advocates the formation of an oligarchy of scientists to rule via "objective" knowledge, is perhaps less the play's hero than its primary hazard. The chapter, and the book, closes with a brief discussion of Hardy's odd novel about free love, *The Well-Beloved*, which was written before his work on *Jude the Obscure* and then rewritten after it, constituting Hardy's own development of his resistance to contemporary biological mandates of purity and isolation. Hardy's surprising insistence on free love in this novel can, I argue, be overlaid against contemporary sewage innovations, as can his insistence on openness and connectivity that was beginning to be discussed in the late century as understanding of probiotics developed.

In focusing on dramatic and fiction-based representations of disease and relationship structures, I hope to focus on the potential of these malleable art forms to explore the limits of human relationships, as well as the boundaries of subjecthood in a diseased world. Because I am less interested in science-making than the cultural effects of science, I have excluded scientific texts from my larger analyses (although they are included as supplements to my readings of fiction). Additionally, while this study covers nineteenth-century British fiction and drama, it also addresses Scandinavian drama. There are a few reasons for this. First, Ibsen's plays burst onto the British literary scene in the late 1880s—precisely the period covered by my project—greatly influencing British literature and culture at this time.[13] Secondly, his plays directly influenced Thomas Hardy, whose fiction is in many ways strikingly similar to Ibsen's drama in terms of its aims and composition dates; in spite of this, almost no work exists connecting the work of these two authors—my fourth and fifth chapters develop this connection. Third, Ibsen expounds upon disease at great length and in many ways much more explicitly than his British counterparts. Finally, the rigidly moralistic society of Norway that Ibsen devoted his work to speaking out against bears many striking resemblances to and illustrates vividly the widespread influence of British Victorian culture, a dynamic that has not been fleshed out in literary studies thus far.[14]

"We Drove in a Body to Science": The Cultural Tides of Nineteenth-Century Scientific Inquiry

Before embarking upon these chapters in their entirety, it is worth taking a moment to consider the general state of the sciences in the Victorian era both before and during germ theory's development. To say that scientific understandings progressed in the nineteenth century is an understatement akin to saying that the invention of the atomic bomb altered warfare. The rapid rate of change across all scientific disciplines, as well as pervasive cultural absorption of these changes, was staggering. From our standpoint in an era when most scientific discoveries are communicated in jargon-laden academic journals accessible neither physically nor intellectually to even a well-educated layman, it is difficult to conceive exactly how staggering these changes were. Nineteenth-century science was indeed explosive, launching into the unknown everything Victorians thought they knew about—the bounds of space, time, the universe itself, and humanity's place in it. Moreover, because scientific studies were less specialized at the time, the average middle- or upper-class reader was well apprised of these developments, which therefore seeped easily into the zeitgeist of the era. The very word *science* is a Victorian invention and did not appear in the OED until 1840.[15] As the findings of William Herschel, Charles Lyell, Charles Darwin, and others like them became widely acknowledged, science, a field that ostensibly aimed to pin down objective knowledge of the world, suddenly seemed to destabilize it, loosing man from his moorings and setting him adrift in the cosmos of destabilized cosmologies.

For example, the overthrow of the biblical timeline of the world's history—made most famous in Charles Lyell's *Principles of Geology*—seemed to stretch the path of history back into an inconceivably long void of prehistory, exposing time as an "abyss"—a looming question mark of unimaginable proportions rather than a comforting and stable presence, populated with known and recognizable characters.[16] In his well-known *Victorian People and Ideas*, Richard Altick describes the schematic adjustment on the collective brains of Victorians as "staggering."[17] His description is apt, as all of the fossils catalogued in Lyell's massive tome, to note one example, seemed not to crystallize a permanent historical narrative, but rather to suggest the impossibility of ever gathering enough specimens to do so and the ultimate unknowability of the bounds of time.[18] Lyell himself lamented the advent of "discoveries which extend indefinitely the bounds of time . . . [and] cause the generations of man to shrink into insignificance and to appear, even when all combined, as ephemeral in duration as the insects which live but from the rising to the setting of the sun."[19] Novelist and scientist alike expressed their existential anxiety in the face of these discoveries—the literal cliffhanger embedded in Thomas Hardy's *A Pair of Blue Eyes* is critically famous today for capturing the layman's response to geological innovation. The protagonist, Henry Knight, a geologist, hangs off the edge of a cliff, holding on for dear life, and yet spends what could be his final living moments in philosophical contemplation of a trilobite fossil he finds himself face-to-face with on the cliff's edge. As he realizes the essential unity of all creatures throughout history in their joint trajectory toward death and decay, "time closed up like a fan before him. He saw himself at one extremity of the years, face to face with the beginning and all the intermediate centuries simultaneously."[20]

The radical shifts in Victorian understanding of the universe were compounded by advances in astronomy. If geology expanded Victorian understanding of time to an unimaginable, yawning abyss, astronomy expanded understanding of space to the extent that man seemed not only an insignificant blip in the geologic strata but also an insignificant speck in an infinite cosmic expanse.[21] In 1831, for instance, Thomas Henderson plotted the distance to the nearest star at 24 trillion miles from the earth.[22] This discovery represents just one example of the sort of astronomical developments underway at this time. The advent of the second law of thermodynamics in the 1850s, which proved (among other things) the eventual heat death of the universe, was no less comforting.[23]

Advances in chemistry and microscope technology allowed scientists to go past measuring and charting stars to analyzing their physical, chemical components using spectroscopy.[24] In fact, it was from this capability that the field of astrophysics began to emerge.[25] The return of Halley's Comet in 1758 instilled Victorians with a confidence that cosmic occurrences were not signs of world events or harbingers of doom but rather calculable, predictable events that could be analyzed by mathematical and scientific measurement.[26] Importantly, the travel of Venus between the sun and the Earth in 1874 and 1882 (which confident astronomers attempted to map, measure, chart, and photograph—all failed efforts) shook this confidence.[27] Thus, the heavenly bodies remained tantalizingly within reach, but often eluded exact scientific comprehension. Moving on from geology, Hardy went on nearly ten years later to explore the existential crises of the casual astronomer. Astronomer Swithin St. Cleeve and his sweetheart Viviette Constantine, protagonists of *Two on a Tower*, spend their evenings in the early part of their romance traversing the starscape together with the telescope Viviette has purchased for Swithin. Hardy describes the simultaneity of the aching beauty and gnawing terror of probing the depths of the heavens too persistently:

> They plunged down to that at other times invisible stellar mul-
> titude in the back rows of the celestial theatre: remote layers
> of constellations whose shapes were new and singular; pretty

twinklers which for infinite ages had spent their beams without calling forth from a single earthly poet a single line, or being able to bestow a ray of comfort on a single benighted trav- eler. . . . Having got closer to immensity than their fellow-crea- tures, they saw at once its beauty and its frightfulness. They more and more felt the contrast between their own tiny magnitudes and those among which they had recklessly plunged, till they were oppressed with the presence of a vastness they could not cope with even as an idea, and which hung about them like a nightmare.[28]

"The presence of a vastness": this is perhaps the most apt way to describe the souvenirs of nineteenth-century scientific fervor. For all their intellectual efforts, busy scientists seem to provide society with the sense of a palpable absence of certainty and a concomitant rendering asunder and snatching away of previous certainties. The only surety left seemed a bleak one indeed: religious discourse seemed consequently but certainly impotent as a means of fully explaining this vast new nature as revealed not by a Messiah, but by science, and science itself provided no new helpful cosmology but merely set society adrift in unnavigable waters, with no compass to point out safe harbors.

Of course, Darwin's theory of evolution is the most famous culprit targeted for secularizing society, as J. Hillis Miller, Gillian Beer, and George Levine—to cite just the most famous examples—have all explored at length. Miller's 1963 study, *The Disappearance of God: Five Nineteenth-Century Writers,* which focuses on secularization more than it does Darwin, remains helpful in distinguishing what is meant by a secular culture, or a culture without God, especially given the undeniable fact that many Victorians continued to identify as Christian in spite of this ostensible secularization.[29] Although it would be impossible to claim that Victorians were by and large atheists, even for those who continued to adhere to the religion nominally or spiritually, "the lines of connection between [man] and God ha[d] broken down . . . God himself has slipped away from the places where he used to be. He no longer inheres in the world as the force binding together all men and all things."[30] This secularization left humankind, content for centuries to rely upon religion as a guiding social force, in a strangely bewildering place, lost in the desert of uncertainty perversely bequeathed to him by science. Or, as Matthew Arnold most aptly put it (and as Miller in fact quotes to this end), Victorian science seemed to jilt society at the altar, bringing humanity to the brink of new understanding, and then leaving him alone to sort out the results for himself—leaving him, as it were, "wandering between two worlds, one dead, / The other powerless to be born."[31] Victorians, then, found themselves alone in a wilderness created by their own intellectual capacity and faced with "the problem of learning to live with and understand" the world around them even while "the God who was thought to have created all that abundance and variety of differences was being expelled."[32]

Germ Theory and the Pursuit of Purity

George Levine asserts that continued scientific inquiry was, paradoxically, one way Victorians navigated the new world in which they had been left adrift by science itself—one way, that is, that they attempted to "know" this world objectively in a time of constantly shifting cosmologies. As he claims in his discussion of Huxley, "scientific knowledge" seemed to be "beyond prejudice, and claim[ed] the authority lost by religion."[33] What I would like to suggest here, however, is that germ theory (which associated one microbe with each illness, rather than citing miasmas, or noxious vapors, as disease vectors) in particular offered Victorian society a form of scientific knowledge that seemed somehow more objective and stable than previous fields of inquiry. Geology had rendered asunder the bowels of the earth, astronomy had opened up the black, gaping maw of the heavens in all its terrifying infinity, and even the history revealed by Darwinian evolution had yanked man from his pedestal as a supremely perfected being, and situated him instead alongside the puny trilobite. Following the frenetic embrace of germ theory in popular culture, the simple and palatable idea that one microbe accompanied one illness washed over society like a soothing bath. The notion that the heretofore spiritually and physically murky realm of death and disease could now be easily grasped, and perhaps one day controlled, came to a society more than willing to accept this palliative as a veritable social panacea. The world seemed on the verge of resituating itself along the teleological path to perfection that Darwin so famously destabilized. And the greater part of Victorian society clung to this potential certainty with a vise-grip of tensile strength possible in only the most existentially anxious. The stranglehold of these axioms—cleanse, purify, sanitize—launched a countercultural movement in literature that the following chapters hone in on. However, this stronghold is no longer obvious to us, both because of our 160-year remove from the cultural tenor of the Victorians, but also because we have simply inherited their attitudes toward germs—as our current struggle with antibiotic-resistant pathogens demonstrates.

Although Pasteur's work with yeast and microbes in France is perhaps the most famous set of early experiments regarding germ theory, similar work was going on throughout Europe, and the findings of all such scientists were published widely. In general, the period of the 1860s and '70s were marked by a decisive move away from a belief in miasma theory to the belief that specific illnesses were caused by unique strains of germs. While variations of germ-based theories of disease had been proposed earlier—indeed, even as early as ancient times—and although groups of people continued to espouse miasma theory into the late nineteenth century, the ten-year period between 1860–1870 marks the main period of experimentation with and popularization of the idea of microbial vectors of disease, after which (in the 1880s and onward) germ theory and bacteriology had decisive hold of popular and scientific culture. In 1861, Ignasz Semmelweis published meticulous treaties on the contagious nature of a specific disease, puerperal fever, and was fired for his writings, but his work contributed generally to the understanding of microbial infection.[34] As will be seen in chapter 2, his work was taken up by a number of physicians in America, including notable thinkers such as Oliver Wendell Holmes.[35] In England, Joseph Lister, whose name is now immortalized in the antiseptic mouthwash Listerine, experimented with wound infections and the antiseptic and aseptic techniques for combatting them.[36] Lister's work, like Semmelweis's, utilized specific examples of infection to promote the idea that microbial agents were involved in infection and could be combatted. A decade or so later, in the 1880s, Robert Koch would rise to fame for his identification of numerous bacterial pathogens, including the vector for the infamous tuberculosis.

After the initial period of experimentation with germ theory in the 1860s and 1870s, the field of bacteriology developed in the 1880s as the source of evidentiary support for the theory. For instance, Pasteur's famous foundational work with yeast and microorganisms in the late 1860s and early 1870s (which proved the existence of organic, growing material in aerobic environments) led to his later work treating rabies and anthrax in the 1880s (after he specifically identified the causative agents associated with these illnesses). More prominent for his bacteriological research specifically, Robert Koch's work with bacteria in the early 1880s led a confident march forward in the scientific profession and the science-consuming public as his experiments bolstered the certainty that all germs could be found, secured

on a microscope slide, and studied.[37] By this time germ theory, now supported by the new field of bacteriology, had gained new fervor. As germ
theory was increasingly the predominant theory used to explain disease,
scientists around the world scrambled to make their name by being the
next hero to identify a virulent pathogen—enter the era of the "Microbe
Hunters."[38] Gone were the days of William Farr's and John Snow's epidemiological maps, which attempted to represent visually the pervasiveness of
poisonous miasmas in order to identify the environments in which disease
festered. The so-called Microbe Hunters of the 1880s became figures of
ever-strengthening centrifugal force as society reveled in its newfound ability
to pinpoint disease vectors.

The Unlike other fields of science, bacteriology seemed to offer stable
knowledge as the germ accompanying each contemporary endemic disease
was discovered and verified. Although most of these discoveries were not
accompanied by cures (rabies and anthrax were two notable exceptions),
bacteriology provided hard evidence of the causes of diseases that had long
plagued and unfortunately continued to plague society. Victorian scientists
and the popular culture at large latched onto this buoy of certainty with
a desperate vise-grip in the wake of the unknowns left to them by previous scientific inquiries in other fields. For Victorians, then, I argue, germ
theory and its sidekick bacteriology were an irresistible promise of ultimate
truth in a world of shifting cosmologies. Furthermore, as I have already
suggested, the Victorian chokehold on the potential truth claims offered by
these fields was that of the desperate soul, clinging to a rocky shore after
months adrift at sea.

The fever pitch of Victorian enthusiasm about germ theory and the
certainty it offered is practically palpable in any periodical publication on
the subject. "The 'germ theory' of disease spread like one of the epidemics which it explained," one article asserts cheerfully, "and revolutionized
half our ideas of disease and treatment . . . [in a] whirlwind of progress."[39]
Another article lauds the efforts of germ theorists, exclaiming that "it is
the noble aim of Science, to be able . . . to keep [disease] under efficient
control."[40] Still other articles reiterate the collective social relief found in
such a certain realm of science whose claims seemed unimpeachable by
the 1880s. Speaking with almost religious fervor, for example, one article
affirms the social support of germ theory, announcing: "[T]oday we pin our
pathological faith on the germ theory, and scientific men the world over are
endeavoring to isolate the specific germ of each particular disease."[41] Another
underscores the certainty afforded by germ theory in its explanation that "the

germ theory is firmly established on the basis of facts that are unassailable, and that are daily receiving new accessions of strength."[42]

Most recent microhistories of germ theory work against the notion that there were any fundamentally new truths discovered with germ theory, or any truly new sights seen, however. That is, germ theory seemingly offered very little that was new or different from previous epistemologies such as miasma theory. Laura Otis notes, for instance, that "many factors besides the essential technical ones affect what one sees under a microscope, or at least the way one describes it," pointing out by way of example that "the realization that microorganisms cause diseases . . . could have easily been made with Leeuwenhoek's lenses in the 1670s."[43] Otis ultimately pinpoints contemporary imperialistic mindsets as shaping broad cultural notions which allowed scientists to "see" microbes for the first time as such:

> Cell theory relies on the ability to perceive borders, for to see a structure under a microscope means to visualize a membrane that distinguishes it from its surroundings. Germ theory, the idea that infectious diseases are caused by living microorganisms, encourages one to think in terms of "inside" and "outside" to an even greater extent.[44]

Otis goes on in subsequent chapters to recast the dynamic between Rudolf Virchow, notoriously labeled "backward" in traditional histories for his ostensible rejection of germ theory, and Koch, typically labeled as a more progressive Microbe Hunter. Otis helpfully points out that Virchow in fact did not deny the physical evidence of microbial existence, but rather believed that the views of germ theory tended to encourage a conservative political agenda that ignored the needs of the lower classes; on the other hand, Otis exposes a counternarrative of Koch's career, highlighting his vocal support of imperialist projects, including forcibly vaccinating colonized groups to cleanse them of diseases that the imperialists feared.[45] "If diseases were associated with the poor rather than poverty itself," Otis argues in summation of Virchow's perspective, "the health of the bourgeoisie might be safeguarded simply by minimizing their contact with the lower classes."[46] Christopher Hamlin has also noted that debates about contagion versus miasma theories "had more to do with politics than with theoretical medicine."[47] Thus, not only were there sociopolitical factors affecting the creation of new scientific understandings, but also, and more importantly for my project, these new scientific epistemologies had vast social implications. "If one believes invisible germs, spread by human contact, can make one sick, one becomes more and more anxious about penetration and about any connection with other people," Otis concludes, a fact she attributes to growing imperialist anxieties in the age of rampant colonialism.[48]

It is perhaps clear by now that my project builds upon the scope of Otis's. Instead of the political forces constructing science, however, I consider here the social impact of extant science; and, instead of focusing on anxieties about contact with foreigners alone, I would like to consider the ways the growing authority of germ theory tended to suggest that any and all contact with others was dangerous and potentially deadly. In a society that had lost its God—at least the God that had once "inhered" in society, as Miller puts it—because of scientific inquiries that exposed the ultimate uncertainty of nature, the scientific and reading public paradoxically turned to germ theory with renewed spiritual vigor for its potential to lay claim to objective truths under the microscope. Germ theory emerged as a new potential Godhead, a new arbiter of behavior, (inter)action, and purity. Along with its ideological imperatives came authors who provocatively argued against aseptic isolation and for the risk that comes along with human encounters.

As Otis has noted, there are few practical differences between the rhetoric of germ and miasma theory. Both suggest that invisible, airborne particles cause disease, and that these particles fester in certain environments, whether filthy alley or Petri dish. Both could offer little more than basic sanitation and hygiene (already available from the previously extant sanitation/hygiene movement) as a curative for cleansing spaces (miasma theory) and people (germ theory). David Barnes summarizes the effects of germ theory's rather unoriginal innovations:

> The germ theory of disease changed everything and nothing at all. . . . In the late 1870s, nearly all medical observers agreed on the fundamental causes of disease: heredity, climate, miasmas, immoderate lifestyles. Some diseases were considered to be contagious in some circumstances—smallpox and syphilis, for example—but even those could usually be traced to these fundamental causes. By the mid-1890s, all but a few holdouts considered living microorganisms the only true cause of infectious disease. . . . The practical strategies recommended for preventing disease, however, had changed little.[49]

Barnes's compelling summary, of course, leads to the question of just what purpose germ theory served socially, if it did not fundamentally alter the means of handling disease—especially since medical treatments for the most common disease culprits such as cholera, typhus, typhoid, syphilis, and tuberculosis were still ephemeral possibilities of the distant future. The answer as I see it brings my introduction full circle: Victorian society treated germ theory as their deliverance from a world void of certainty, as the source of manageable, certain, and objective knowledge. This new movement

> made possible a new way of understanding, explaining, and combating disease in society by integrating the old concerns of the sanitary movement (filth and contamination, cleanliness and morality) with a new germ-centered focus on the danger of contact with potentially sick bodies and bodily substances, tests for the presence of microbes, and the promise of their control through laboratory science. . . . In the age of the sanitary-biological synthesis, filth still causes disease (as it always did), but only science can identify it, explain it, and cure it.[50]

Levine has pointed out in his discussions of Victorian secularization and moral wandering that the old adage "goodness is truth, truth goodness. . . . is a very Victorian notion" that "runs deep" (vi). However, he adds, "it also runs into trouble very quickly" when explored in the face of Victorian uncertainty of what exactly truth *was*.[51] In the late-century context where germ theory had become the increasingly authoritative neonate-God of a world "struggling to be born" and had been bolstered by the already-extant practices of the sanitary movement alongside the burgeoning field of bacteriology, it finally seemed possible to grasp the "good" through "proper" sanitation practices. Health and freedom from disease, it seemed, was at least one way of establishing some sure footing on the path toward social and personal progress.

Barnes provides countless examples of attempts to literally scrub the detritus of the world out of the common man's existence, as if clearing away microbes that threatened bare life could simultaneously clear the existential doubt that marked so much of Victorian existential crisis. In Paris, trucks were established to go into the homes of the previously sick and sanitize them to perfection. Barnes quotes a 1901 disinfection procedure invoked by such technicians:

For residential disinfections, we follow the following rules: upon departing the station, each vehicle is accompanied by a coachman and two disinfectors. The wagons are enclosed, with smooth, *impermeable* interior surfaces. . . . With the hose spraying disinfectant liquid, the agents begin by dampening one area, then they install in that area the packages, cloth covers, or baskets and place there (after folding them carefully) all objects capable of being taken to the *disinfection tank*. Packages must be *hermetically sealed*. They then proceed to disinfect the rooms and furniture by spraying the liquid [containing the] pulverized disinfectant on the walls, the ceilings, the paneling, the floors.[52]

In the desperate push for some epistemological certainty, Victorians solidified the cultural sense that absolute purity was possible to attain and indeed to *main*tain if one could only be thorough enough. The belief in the possibility of completely impermeable surfaces—the idea that "carefully" packaged household items could be "hermetically sealed" and carried to an equally impenetrable "disinfection tank" without cross-contamination taking place—would certainly be a reassuring one even today. In microbial purity, it seemed there could be some certainty in the universe. Bacteriology offered up for viewing and analysis a world quite different from the vast, gaping sinkholes of uncertainty opened by other fields of science. Here, with the microscope, was certain wisdom: carefully comply with a set of rules and man will be superior to disease. The previously cited instructional account goes on to advise that every object in the home must be sprayed down carefully—even the undersides of beds and the backs of paintings—and it describes the proper method of "methodical" coverage using a spray hose to ensure absolute saturation with disinfectant.[53] After adequate disinfection, the manual continues, the bodies of the technicians must be carefully sprayed down "top to bottom," after which the technicians transport the hermetically sealed packages of household goods back to the disinfecting station.[54] From here, the items are transferred via an elaborate conveyance process through sealed chambers within a disinfectant tank so as to allow no contact with the outside world until decontamination with steam is complete.

Such measures in Paris were not simply extreme examples. After the establishment of public disinfection crews in 1889, the city operated four such disinfection stations and "performed thousands of operations in homes throughout the city every year."[55] Of course, although the instructional description claims that "after a certain amount of practice, disinfection" of a person's home "can be easily done without subjecting the objects undergoing it to any deterioration," another facet of this process was obviously its public reception.[56] As Barnes points out through a series of extended examples in his monograph, although some people balked at the damage to their items, most seemed increasingly willing to undergo this process for the sake of a belief in the total purity of their homes and their bodies. As Barnes notes, though, "the stigma and intrusiveness" of disinfection "did not disappear" entirely.[57] As it "gained in familiarity and popularity . . . [it] succeeded . . . in subtly altering individual and collective expectations" of the potential for and propriety of perfect antisepsis.[58] Similar purification methods were used in Britain, as well. A letter on "Successful Disinfection" written by the Medical Officer of Health for Bristol in 1867 offers a similar plan of disinfection:

> The city is divided into four districts; each district has an inspector in it, there is also a superintendent inspector; each district inspector in the summer time has two workmen at his command, and one in the winter, to white-lime dirty walls, courts, and alleys. . . . They carry with them a bucket of [disinfecting powder] which they sprinkle over the pans . . . of the closets, over every street grating and every eject they pass. When we suspect any division of the sewers to have the germs of disease in it, we throw in a considerable quantity. . . . I meet the district inspectors daily at 11 a.m., and if they report any disease of a zymotic character among the poor, I visit the affected persons and order the floor to be thickly sprinkled with [the] powder. If the patient dies, or is removed, we supply some to be sprinkled over the corpse.[59]

Barnes's assertion is clearly accurate, as, in spite of Victorian norms and propriety surrounding respect for the dead, which included elaborate means of preserving and revering the body itself, seemingly the population spoken of here ostensibly willingly allowed dubious substances to be poured on the bodies of their departed family members.

This drive for purity can be found throughout a range of Victorian periodicals. One article concludes by explaining that "*pure* air, or air as free from destructive germs as can be procured, is now felt to be one of the first considerations in choosing a dwelling, and in getting out of the way of noxious impurities."[60] Another article instructs readers, in rather as much detail as Barnes's previously cited tract, about maintaining the purity of a sickroom, or at least hermetically isolating its infectious particles within it. "It can readily be seen," the article proclaims confidently,

> that anything that will kill the germs, and prevent their absorp-
> tion and multiplication will limit the disease. For this use the
> room should be uncarpeted and all woolen articles, as tending
> to absorb the poisonous elements, should be removed from it;
> the brooms and cloths used in collecting the dust should not
> be taken to any other part of the house, and all clothing or
> bedding should be thoroughly disinfected before taken to the
> wash. Corrosive sublimate 1 part to 1,000 of water, is one of
> the best solutions for the purpose.[61]

The author continues to describe methods of maintaining a hermetically sealed room of contagion: "[T]he room must be tightly closed, all cracks around doors and windows filled with cotton, and thoroughly fumigated with Sulphur."[62] Aside from domestic instruction guides, advertisements of the time capitalized on the Victorian obsession with purification. A late-century advertisement for the heavily marketed Izal Powder relies on the rhetoric of purity and faith in aseptic possibilities (see Figure I.1).[63] The two-page advertisement proclaims the product's wonders, describing "its extraordinary antiseptic potency," and adding that the product boasts "the fullest confirmation from the highest sanitary authorities of the day."[64]

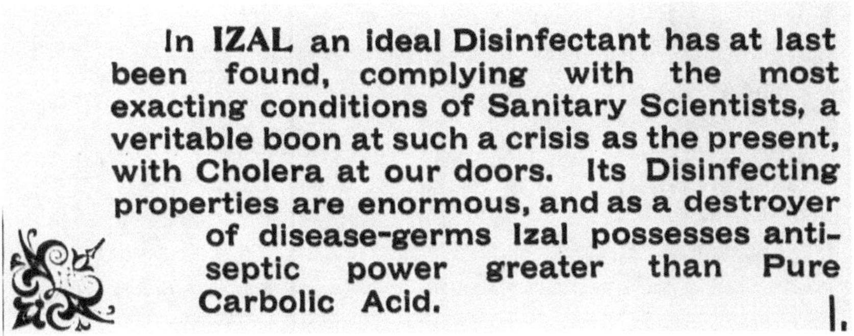

In IZAL an ideal Disinfectant has at last been found, complying with the most exacting conditions of Sanitary Scientists, a veritable boon at such a crisis as the present, with Cholera at our doors. Its Disinfecting properties are enormous, and as a destroyer of disease-germs Izal possesses antiseptic power greater than Pure Carbolic Acid. **I.**

Figure I.1. Advertisement for Izal Disinfectant, 1893.

An advertisement for Eno's Fruit Salt proclaims that the nation as a whole can be purified through collective use of the blood-cleansing product (see Figure I.2).[65] Aside from relying on nationalistic rhetoric, the advertisement makes full use of the public's preoccupation with microbial purity, boasting that "you cannot overstate its great value in keeping the blood pure and free from disease."[66] "Blood cleansers" were in fact all the rage in late Victorian England. These products built upon the broad social sense that perfect purity is both achievable and desirable, and, similar to domestic instruction guides, operated upon the notion that impurities are vulnerable to the effects of cleaning, scrubbing, or washing, rather than allowing for their organic state. Another blood cleanser, Clarke's brand, proclaims that it is "warranted to cleanse the blood from all impurities from *whatever* cause arising," and warns readers to "beware of worthless imitations."[67] Carbolic smoke balls were popular products, built upon notions of disinfection by implying that its vapor-based disinfectant allows its purifying effects to penetrate all cells of the body when inhaled (see Figures I.3 and I.4).[68] Another Eno's Fruit

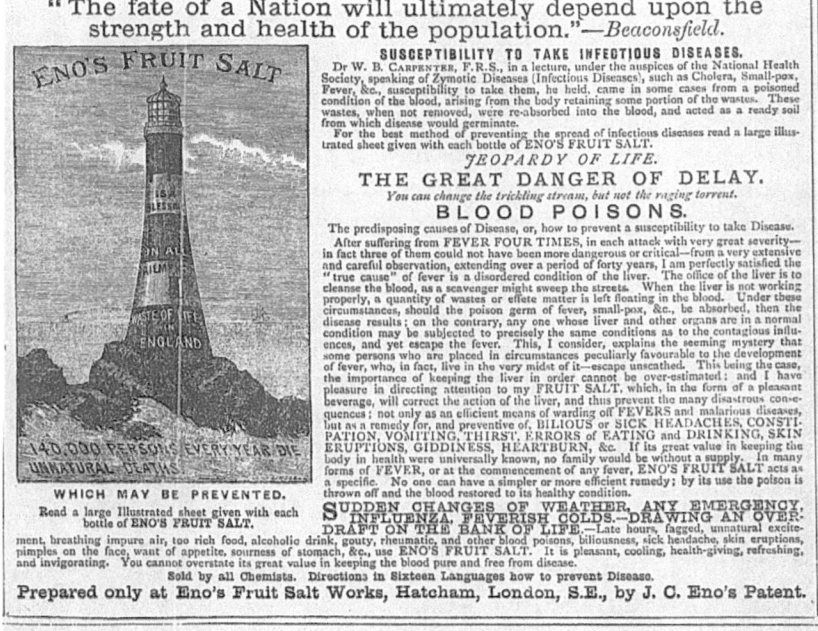

Figure I.2. Advertisement for Eno's Fruit Salt, 1897.

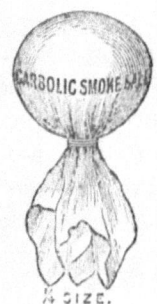

FREE TRIALS TO ALL,

AT OUR OFFICES, 202, REGENT ST.

THE CARBOLIC SMOKE BALL

WILL POSITIVELY CURE

CATARRH,   PNEUMONIA,   THROAT DEAFNESS,
ASTHMA,   NEURALGIA,   CROUP,
BRONCHITIS,   LOSS OF VOICE,   HAY FEVER,
      COUGHS, COLDS, and all troubles caused by taking cold.
                    FOR INHALATION ONLY.
       One Smoke Ball will last a family from six months to one year. Thus it
is the cheapest remedy in the world. It will be sent, post free, with full
directions for use, on receipt of the price, 10s. Address:—

Carbolic Smoke Ball Co., 202, Regent-st., London, W.

Figure I.3. Advertisement for Carbolic Smoke Ball, 1889.

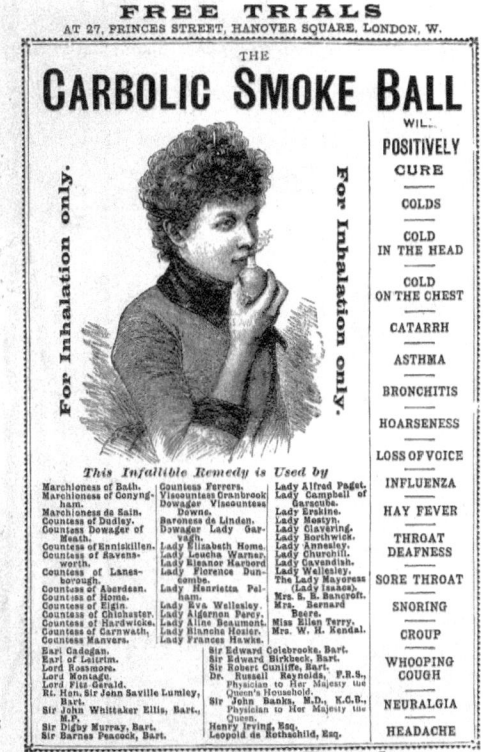

Figure I.4. Advertisement for Carbolic Smoke Ball, 1890.

Salt ad draws upon this notion of the necessity of perfect purification of the air by describing the skin itself as "an everted lung."[69] This image of an internal organ exposed to the outward atmosphere, rather than maintained in the hermetic seal of our own bodily envelopes, and thus in need of sanitization, is quite typical of the ideological aims of germ theory–based product marketing in this period. Just as advertisers capitalized on the notion of the possibilities of completely cleansing each and every blood cell, atmospheric purifiers such as these built upon the idea that cleansing every molecule of air was both possible and desirable. Carbolic acid was one commonly known and readily available antiseptic, and many products marketed its use in households. The product shown in Figures I.5 and I.6 operates on a relatively common design involving heating a sample of carbolic acid for diffusion into a room. This particular specimen goes so far as to discuss germ theory at length on the box, building the authoritative heft of scientific discourse into its very packaging. In fact, three of the four largest sides of the box are covered in scientific discourse promoting the product's

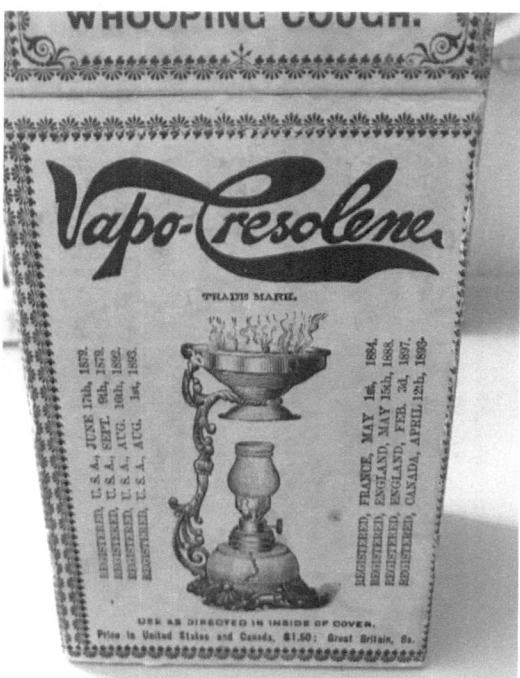

Figure I.5. Product Packaging for Vapo-Cresolene Antiseptic Vapor Diffuser.

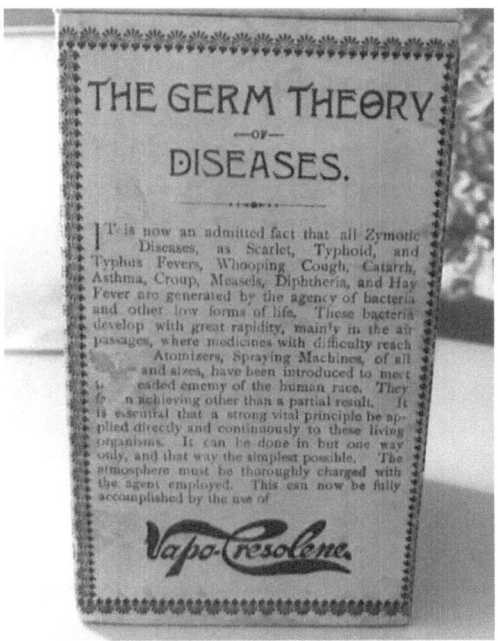

Figure I.6. Product Packaging for Vapo-Cresolene Antiseptic Vapor Diffuser.

efficacy. Another side touts the product's antiseptic abilities, asserting that "vaporizing" of disinfectant substances

> is the true system of disseminating healing . . . agents through the atmosphere; the air is completely charged with the very essence of the compound used. Every crevice is reached. Carpets, Clothing and bedding, a common medium for conveying infection, are purified, the air passages and lungs of the patient are penetrated, and the restorative vapor touches every part.[70]

Of course, as Otis and others have noted, and as I have already mentioned, there were obviously those who did not unequivocally accept germ theory's new authority. Indeed, Martin Willis has discussed at length the interesting fact that Victorians often did not tacitly accept supposedly "objective" visual data seen through a microscope as pure truth, but rather acknowledged the ultimate subjectivity of all visual perception, even that which fell under the realm of "authoritative" science. To cite one additional example, Florence Nightingale has long been critically acknowledged as one of the late holdouts in support of miasma theory who saw little use for germ theory. Like Virchow, however, it appears that her disavowal of the new mode of disease conceptualization had at least as much to do with the social implications of germ theory as with any actual disbelief in its veracity. And yet, Barnes is correct in his general assertion that by the turn of the century, "all but a few holdouts" believed in the general truth claims of germ theory and bacteriology.[71] As his examples show, the general faith in the promise of bacteriology can be easily seen in the great lengths people went to in order to disinfect their world as the sanitary movement was now undergirded by the authoritative heft of germ theory. As he notes, "the case for disinfection could [now] be made on specific scientific grounds" that seemed more certain—especially to a society desperate for some sort of certainty—than previous appeals to mere cleanliness.[72]

Even today, the only thing as dependable as death and taxes is disease. Any person claiming to live an entire life without contracting a communicable illness purports to boast both a genetically impenetrable immune system and the ability to avoid the invisible ephemera we call "germs." Such a superhuman has yet to exist. Indeed, the whole of the human race has been invisibly sculpted by the lives of bacteria, who make their paths in life by eating their way through ours, or (as we now know) often by living in wondrous symbiosis within our bodies. Equal numbers of viruses—those ghostly shades hovering in the liminal space between life and death—have reprogrammed human bodies, resulting in epidemics, pandemics, and hysteria.

Death can be peaceful. Taxes serve certain social functions. But contagious disease is notoriously and intractably messy. Its presence is denoted by all against which we revolt: blood, pus, phlegm, boils. To become diseased is to know that one's body has been infiltrated by an army that cannot be fought. Even in the age of antibiotics and antiviral medicines, the ill individual has no voluntary post hoc defenses against disease. Disease remains that which renders the human body physically helpless, the mind prone and defeated, and the soul disillusioned and in search of purpose amid tragedy. The Victorians—the very first social group to encounter (conceptually) the vast wealth of illnesses as communicable—constitute a helpful case study in beginning to understand our own relationship to disease, interactions that are often as socially and politically shaped as they are biologically and epidemiologically. The swift isolation of Ebola in America in September 2014 compared with its rampant, uncontrolled spread in Africa is one stark example of the social and economic factors—such as access to care and the remaining legacy of colonial dominion—that impact disease in ways less comfortable for us to digest than the purely factual aspects of its virulence, a point to which I will return in my conclusion.

Ultimately, this book asks readers to consider the ways we might develop our own understanding of disease by understanding the Victorians' awe-filled first encounter with epidemiology as we understand it today. For instance, in what ways could we benefit from some of the latest Victorians' claims that science does not have all the answers? Or, at the very least, what might we gain from a consideration of Victorian authors' convictions that science's answers are often vitiating, rather than empowering, and that there is more to vitality than *biological* vitality? How might an understanding of something beyond the bare life expand our notions of end-of-life experiences and terminal diseases? In what ways has an unthinking faith in the new creed of science robbed us today of the potential of a human-centered world that relies not on external validation of reified bioepidemiological factors but on connection with our fellow man, and a humanitarian focus that this connection would allow for? What if we were open to risky encounters with the dangerous but enlightening world around us?

There is much of value in the real and aching struggle of Victorians to achieve a unity of experience and human connection to their fellow man, though it was an oftentimes scary and threatening journey through foul miasmas and festering germs alike. The authors covered here vocalized and dramatized this imperative most fully by underscoring over and over in their fictional creations the notion that engagement in the world is necessary for collective self-actualized existence. That is, late-Victorian authors across continents and cultures repeatedly suggested that a life lived alone is no life. I argue that their alternative—clearly depicted throughout their fictional worlds—reveals that it is better to live in the world, to engage in what I call "risk encounters" with the messy conglomeration of other bodies that populate it, than to stagnate in isolation, dominated and sequestered by the new social arbiter of germ theory–based science.

Keep Bleeding

Plague, Vaccination Debates, and the Necessity of Leaky Boundaries in Defoe's *Journal of the Plague Year* and Shelley's *The Last Man*

How can I be without border? That elsewhere that I imagine beyond the present . . . —it is now here. . . . I behold the breaking down of a world that has erased its borders.

—Julia Kristeva, *Powers of Horror: An Essay on Abjection*

What a sink and receptacle of filth is the body of man? How is he to be restored but by cleansing and purging off the noxious slime and corroded juices which are dispersed in all the vessels of the body, even those vessels which common cathartics will not reach?

—Daniel Defoe, *Journal of the Plague Year*

I begin my consideration of late Victorian reception of germ theory in the early eighteenth century—paradoxical, perhaps. However, just as Freud did not invent, ex nihlio, the concept of divining subconscious desires from dreams, but rather publicized and promoted age-old traditions of dream interpretation, germ theory did not present an absolutely original perspective in its claims that disease could be communicable. The Victorians themselves were quite aware of this. As W. B. Carpenter explains in an 1884 essay on germ theory:

> The idea that such diseases as Small-pox, which spread by human communication, and of which the virus multiplies itself in the human body, are generated by a *contagion vivum* of some kind, is by no means a new one. . . . These general relations were brought out with great force more than forty years ago, by one of our most philosophic physicians, the late Sir Henry Holland, in a thoughtful chapter of his "Medical Notes and Reflections"; but it is only now that their true meaning is becoming apparent in the clear light of the doctrine of disease-germs.[1]

Rather, much like Freud's impact on dream interpretation, germ theory—and, importantly, its latter evidentiary balustrade, bacteriology—popularized rather than invented the concept of communicable disease, making it a commonplace concept as it vastly expanded the realm of exactly what was considered communicable. As Carpenter notes, certain diseases were long known to be contagious. And although Carpenter cites an understanding of contagious diseases from only a half-century before his article, smallpox inoculation began in the 1700s and developed out of an already extant awareness that the illness could be contagious. As an obvious risk encounter involving willingly inserting infected particulates into one's own body to ward off disease, inoculation and the later, Jennerized method of vaccination were controversial from their first introduction into Western society.[2] For its part, plague was far too rampant and far too virulent to avoid widespread identification as contagious; its communicability was simply visible and obvious to even casual observers much before the advent of the scientific method. Germ theory simply broadened the notion of contagion to incorporate an entire set of illnesses, such that today we hardly consider individual systemic complications—heart issues, stroke, anemia, and the like—the same sort of categorical "sickness" as, say, cholera, staphylococcus, or the common cold. Before exploring in detail the ways the conceptual shift ushered in by germ theory affected community relationships and their depiction in fiction, I therefore consider earlier treatment of epidemic plagues as a means by which to hone in on isolated reactions to contagion throughout time. The present analysis foregrounds the concerns of the coming chapters, then, by identifying the specific context of epidemics as a communal condition out of which biopolitical concerns tended to emerge in literature. In demonstrating the knee-jerk isolationist responses that contagious disease tended to catalyze (even before germ theory) and the literary response to it, this chapter thus lays the groundwork for my further arguments about communities in times of disease when the very notion of contagion expanded rapidly in the late nineteenth century.

In this chapter, I read two apocalyptic plague narratives, Daniel Defoe's 1722 *A Journal of the Plague Year* and Mary Shelley's 1826 *The Last Man*, in exploration of literature's capacity to question the superficial borders between the national subject and the international other, alongside the dubious boundary between the self and all that lies outside of it. I overlay these pre-germ-theory contagion narratives with their nearly simultaneous debates regarding inoculation and vaccination, respectively. These debates are important to begin with for several reasons. First, their dependence on disease cosmologies makes them a relevant precursor to the later germ theory of disease, particularly as inoculation developed into vaccination and became valorized as a product of Western medicine and Jenner's genius. Secondly, the debates were both widely read in print and incredibly emotional, because inoculations/vaccinations, by definition, are risk encounters in a quite literal way. As such, these debates and their development encapsulate neatly many of the concerns which I see as becoming pervasive along with germ theory's prevalence.

Horrifying Tokens:
Leaking Sores in *A Journal of the Plague Year*

Defoe's attitude toward infectious plague hearkens to a larger ideology of community as he incorporates into his prescriptive measures economic, medical, and social discourses. Through interpretation of the container of plague contagion, the bubo, this chapter examines Defoe's critique of problematic, isolating public health policies and their effect on community resilience during times of disaster, when Defoe argues this resilience is of the utmost importance. Defoe ultimately advocates permeable interpersonal and national borders that reinforce the vitalizing power of community interaction even in response to the hugely threatening potential of fatal, communicable disease. I argue that Defoe's conceptualization of international trade thoroughly influenced this depiction, which resisted the nationalistic xenophobia typical of his day and instead embraced a type of individualistic mercantilism. Defoe's views on economics and trade, then, influenced his understanding of the Great Plague and cycled back to result in a view of man and nation that advocates permeable boundaries and humanitarianism even in response to the hugely threatening potential of a complete breakdown of self- and nation-constituting borders.[3]

When he is not charting mortality statistics, counting up corpses as they accrue in the plague-infested streets, H. F., the narrator of Daniel Defoe's 1722 *A Journal of the Plague Year*, focuses on the other signifier of the bubonic plague—the eponymous buboes, or pus-filled sores, that characterize the infection. The horrified responses to these indicators of infection pervade the text, and even individuals who are not directly infected often react with existential terror at the sight of them. In one case, H. F. recounts the story of a young mother who, after putting her daughter to bed, "discover[s] the fatal tokens on the inside of her [daughter's] thighs."[4] The discovery of disease within her family is too much to bear:

> Not being able to contain herself, [she] threw down her candle, and shriekt out in such a frightful Manner, that it was enough to place Horror upon the stoutest Heart in the World; nor was it one Skream, or one Cry, but the Fright having seiz'd her Spirits, she fainted first, then recovered, then ran all over the House, up the Stairs and down the Stairs, like one distracted, and indeed really was distracted, and continued screeching and crying out for several Hours, void of all Sense . . . and . . . never came thoroughly to herself again.[5]

The mother loses her own subjectivity at this moment, as the narrator observes that she is never "her*self*" again. Her frenzied, aimless trek through her house, running up the stairs and back down as she screams over and over again, marks her besieged sense of selfhood after merely bearing witness to her daughter's illness.

Defoe's fictive example illustrates vividly here—as Kristeva would go on centuries later to describe in a more theoretical sense—that the difference between oneself and another individual, a component critical to the formation of selfhood, is hardly a demarcation created and maintained in a vacuum. As both authors show in their respective genres, the physical limits of our own bodies—that all-important boundary that separates the precious self within from the messiness without—are of vital importance to this interpersonally constructed subjectivity. And when contagious disease is added to this psycho-physiological cocktail, it reveals the inescapable permeability of cutaneous membranes. In this context, the rules of the subjectivity game suddenly seem less stable, leaving the individual in search of selfhood facing the question, much as the mother does in Defoe's narrative, of how to *be* without borders. As Defoe indicates, the experience of psychic horror in the face of our own physical penetrability is not limited to contact with strangers—the mother in this example panics in the face of her daughter's infective potential. Disease has pierced through the flimsy flesh supposedly protecting her family from the infected, and her psyche crumbles under the weight of the realization that she and those she loves have always been more enmeshed in the messy amalgam of humanity than she had previously dared to believe. Disease has rendered her, as it threatens to render each of us, without borders, defenseless and prone.

Through an exploration of the interpersonal cutaneous borders threatened by disease, this chapter probes the border between the national subject and the international other as well as the boundary between the self and all that lies outside of it. Ultimately, I assert that these two borders are largely intertwined, particularly when considering infectious diseases. The last ten years have seen the advent and dissipation of the threat of numerous potential epidemics—severe acute respiratory syndrome (SARS), the avian flu, and H1N1 influenza, to name only a few. Contagious diseases such as these threaten all subjects with the potential permeation of their bodily envelope by something emitted from other bodies. As Priscilla Wald notes in her compelling book, *Contagious: Cultures, Carriers, and the Outbreak Narrative*, "Disease emergence dramatizes the dilemma that inspires the most basic of human narratives: the necessity and danger of human contact."[6] Illustrating this point quite aptly, scientists ultimately classified each of the diseases listed above as issuing from some *other* (i.e., Eastern) nation. This epidemiological act, while legitimated by contemporary scientific authority, nevertheless continues an age-old Western pattern of situating disease and filth in the realm of anything but the Western self-as-individual or self-as-national-citizen, thereby raising the question of just what ideological ends such ostensibly objective epidemiology serves. Importantly, *A Journal of the Plague Year* makes it abundantly clear that neither threats of disease nor the biased responses to them on the part of both nations and individuals are anything new and that the desire to situate the source of a disease away from one's own identity (both individual and national) is all too representative of the self-interested human condition.

Jennifer Cooke describes the buboes in *A Journal of the Plague Year* as having a "noisy physicality."[7] Indeed, *A Journal of the Plague Year* is a prime example of our psychological and social reliance on protective borders that seem to harbor us and keep us safe from other individuals and nations—the leaky, pus-filled, swollen sores that Defoe defines as the typical "tokens" of the bubonic plague are the Kristevan abject writ large. These oozing pustules, as depicted in the text, illustrate the horror with which people tend to react when the illusory borders they rely on for a sense of personal, social, and national identity break down. The petechiae bruises that give the black plague its nickname, for example, are essentially spots of damaged, injured flesh, and the buboes that give the plague its other colloquial term certainly look like dying, rotting flesh. Both are thus visual representations of each individual's potential to "un-*be*." One's consciousness must jettison this potential in order to maintain a stable sense of selfhood—"in order to live" as a subject.[8] Thus, buboes, the leaky, oozing manifestations of a parasitic life pervading a host life, represent, first, unwanted life, which in attaching itself to and within the host represents a form of the abject literally embodied in and oozing forth from the subject. They also represent a sickening surfeit of fertility, which feeds upon the subject as it proliferates its abject materiality, defying both the subject and those in the subject's company to deny ("to spit out, to eject," as Kristeva would have it) its presence.[9]

Importantly, buboes do more than simply fester as a representation of death literally attached to life. About seven days after infection, buboes usually burst open, spewing their vile and threatening contents forth.[10] The problem with contagion and contaminants, of course, is not simply their symbolic representation of our mortality, but also that these foreign, evasive elements physically break down the illusory border between the self and other necessary for subjectivity. Throughout *A Journal of the Plague Year*, individuals react to the bursting, suppurated buboes with a sense of horror—even those who are presently uninfected—because the visual representation of literally perforated personal borders as seen in the suppurated bubo links even the currently uninfected to the infected in a *community of contagion*.[11]

Certainly, disease is the archetype of that which threatens individual identity and national structural integrity through its pure omnipresence, for even before the advent of germ theory as we conceptualize it today, notions of "foul effluvia" or "odious miasmatic" gases operated upon a similar con-figuration of disease depicted as that which floats blithely and invisibly in the air, no matter its source. Even in 1722, Defoe was certain in his belief that the bubonic plague was contagious, though in regard to its mode of transmission, "whether by effluvia from their bodies, by animalcula mixed and drawn into our bodies with our breath, or by the venom of the tumours, blains, and sores" he acknowledged uncertainty.[12] Thus, in bursting open, suppurated bubonic sores constitute both an involuntary union with others that dissolves any notion of individual selfhood, and also a veritable rape of one's bodily envelope by contagious agents as betokened by the hemorrhagic sore. Trapped as they are in communion with this pathogen, the plague ties the residents of London to one another inextricably and involuntarily, and the important boundaries between the self and the not-self begin to dissolve on individual and aggregate levels. The physical "token" of the buboes, as Defoe repeatedly terms it, strips the individuals who bear them and the individuals who witness them of their individual identity, linking them forcibly into a community conferred upon them only through the binding net of contagious forces.

These leaky sores threaten to literally permeate the boundaries of the individual body and figuratively dissolve the functionality of the nation. Given how important notions of borders seem to be to our maintenance of some idea of selfhood, there is a curious supernumerary character in this text: the *un*suppurated sores, which are given as much, if not more, textual space than the suppurated sores, and which the individuals narrating and depicted in the text, in fact, treat with a great deal *more* anxiety than bursting buboes. Since perforated cutaneous membranes threaten society at large through the very fact of their leakiness, the extreme anxiety with which individuals in *A Journal of the Plague Year* treat *calciferous* buboes is quite curious. Defoe describes the variations of buboes by writing that, in some cases, when the "swellings which were generally in the Neck or Groin" proceeded to become "hard and would not break, [they] grew so painful that it was equal to the most exquisite Torture."[13] According to Defoe,

> The pain of the swelling was in particular very violent, and to some intolerable; the physicians and surgeons may be said to have tortured many poor creatures, even to death. The swellings in some grew hard, and they apply'd violent drawing plasters, or poultices, to break them; and if these did not do, they cut and scarified them in a terrible manner: In some, those swellings were made hard, partly by the force of the distemper, and partly by their being too violently drawn, and were so hard that no instrument could cut them, and then they burnt them with causticks, so that many died raving mad with the torment; and some in the very operation.[14]

In the case of one man in particular, whose buboes "cou'd not be brought to break, or to suppurate . . . the Surgeons had, it seems, hopes to break them, which Causticks were [for that reason] then upon him, burning his Flesh as with a hot Iron."[15] If the leaky, suppurated sores typical of the bubonic plague are so threatening to all forms of identity, it would seem that hardened sores that refuse to burst represent a safely quarantined storehouse of contagion. Why, then, the determined efforts to force these sores to burst? Rather than regard them as a realm of safely quarantined contagion, doctors voraciously attack the hardened buboes in this text, piercing, prodding, and forcing them to climactic emission against all odds. Here, I would argue, Defoe creates a risk encounter, forcibly depicting the tearing down of these boundaries, so intent is he on the value of these exposures. The determined doctors seem oddly intent on this necessity, even resorting, as Defoe notes, to the "torture" of "many poor creatures."[16] Defoe's repeated depictions of the violent efforts to force the suppuration of hardened sores demonstrate his firm belief that a mediated, controlled flow of all things was the only viable response to the plague. His value of these risk encounters—such that he repeatedly depicts their *creation* of a risky border where one was not previously present—is, among other things, influenced by his personal theories of economics and trade, all of which advocated an individualistic mercantilism.

A Hard Pill to Swallow:
Risk Encounters, Inoculation, and Identity

It is worth mentioning here that while many critics ascribe the advent of *A Journal of a Plague Year* to the plague outbreak that had arisen in Europe in the early 1720s and seemed likely to enter London, I would argue that more than just contemporary plague outbreaks could account for the composition of this text. This is not to deny, of course, the relevance a publication such as Defoe's would have undoubtedly had in the context of an impending plague epidemic within London. However, another outbreak in this same period, one that took place within the very confines of the city itself, has been relatively neglected in critical consideration of *A Journal*'s publication. In 1721, a smallpox epidemic beset London.[17] This outbreak provoked eighteenth-century scientists in England to experiment with variolation using the smallpox virus.[18] It is important to note to this end that *A Journal* is not Defoe's first foray into plague writings. Defoe had published multiple, smaller tracts on the subject for nearly a decade by the 1720s.[19] That his most extensive texts on the subject, *A Journal of the Plague Year* and *Due Preparations for the Plague*, were published only a year after this local outbreak of smallpox is a point of fact that is problematic to ignore. It would seem that this actual and local smallpox epidemic must have also influenced Defoe's composition of these works at least as much as a distant outbreak of the plague that might not reach London.

Wald notes that "outbreak narratives proliferate in periods of major demographic shifts and increased social contact."[20] The smallpox epidemic initiated a fear not just of the contagious other but also of incorporating the other into the self. Inoculation involves depositing a small amount of infected matter from the sore of an individual infected with smallpox into a purposely inflicted wound located on the body of a healthy person. Thus, contemporary smallpox inoculation essentially involved a voluntary acceptance of the diseased other into the material body of the self as a prophylactic measure against actually *becoming* a part of this contagious threat. While many saw such an act as necessary to the preservation of life, the traumatic potential of laying aside self-constituting psychic boundaries for the sake of preservation of bare life should by now be clear. The public debates about inoculation were accordingly passionate.[21] A 1730 tract opens by acknowledging the well-recognized and long-standing nature of the debates, as well as their emotional character:

> [T]here have been too early and strong prejudices, both for and against this method; people have been partially credulous or incredulous of facts, as they make for or against their respective opinions, viz, in some it favoured much of credulity, levity, and novelty, to be bigotly zealous for it; in others, it show'd too much of strong prejudices, passions or obstinate humour, to be furiously against it.[22]

Writing some years after Defoe's text, William Douglass tracks the earlier history (contemporary with *A Journal of the Plague Year*) of the techne. Though Douglass is ultimately a proponent of inoculation, he addresses the legitimate early concerns with secondary infections from inoculation when the practice was being learned in England. He states:

> We find by some years experience, that the Small Pox abstractedly considered, received by inoculation is not so fatal and the symptoms frequently more miled, than in the accidental contagion; yet it is not of that certain safety, to exempt it from being reckoned precarious, and therefore requires discretion in applying it to proper subjects, and judgment in managing the distemper so received.[23]

Indeed, early attempts at inoculation, imperfectly reproduced in Britain, could be dangerous. An earlier 1722 tract bears in its very title the emotional verve of the inoculation debates that Douglass recounts. Legard Sparham's *Reasons against the Practice of Inoculating the Small-Pox as also A Brief Account of the Operation of This Poison, Infused after This Manner into a Wound*, is a typical example of these proto-"anti-vaxx" pamphlets.[24] Sparham bemoans "the instilling of poison into a wound," which, as he argues, is so widely "accounted the most destructive of any" practice. The suppuration of a skin barrier and the incorporation of "a fermented matter admitted into the blood by a sore" bypasses, to his mind, all the body's natural defenses in a ghastly manner.[25]

During this time, then, society at large was tasked with an existential paradox: in order to prevent a complete breakdown between the self and the other in the midst of the community of contagion, the only choice available to those living amid the smallpox epidemic was inoculation. And yet, as another 1722 treatise expounds, this conscientious choice is simply counterintuitive. "If we consult our reason and experience as to" inoculation, W. Wagstaffe states, "we shall scarcely find it sufficient to answer [the] purpose."[26] He continues his argument alongside a description of inoculation, noting that "the very choice that is made of a thick purulent matter to intermix immediately with the blood, seems a little repugnant to our reason."[27] Allowing for the transmission of a slight bit of matter from the other into the self prevented the complete parasitic takeover by this ever-threatening other. Thus, to preserve bare, physical life and avoid a complete psychological breakdown of the self through uncontrolled, suppurated sores, individuals willing to engage with risk encounters opted to maintain the ultimate viability of these barriers (both physical and mental) by temporarily allowing for the moderate, controlled permeation of these boundaries.

The hardened sores, in bringing about such fervent efforts to penetrate their boundaries, illustrate clearly how influenced Defoe was by the need for the controlled, mediated permeation of boundaries he saw in the inoculative response to smallpox. Granted, the bubonic plague is not a disease that can be inoculated against. Even in Defoe's own age one of the few things the public knew for certain about the plague was that having the disease did not preclude the possibility of contracting it again, which would have rendered it an unlikely candidate for attempts at inoculation.[28] Nevertheless, the concept of inoculation—taking a bit of the threatening other into the self as a prophylactic measure against a complete takeover by this other—clearly influenced Defoe's views in handling the practical effects of the plague after the 1721 smallpox outbreak.

The epidemics in and around London and England just prior to the publication of his text undoubtedly influenced Defoe. Of course, Defoe's ever-apparent fiscal pragmatism is also integral to this work. Even amid the trauma of the plague, trade worms its way into the narrative of *A Journal.*[29] H. F. is at great pains to account for the precise loss to trade effected by the plague. Even during the early inception of the plague into the body of London, H. F. notes that "from that Hour, all Trade, except such as related to immediate Subsistence, was, *as it were,* at a full Stop."[30] Meaning here domestic trade, H. F. then goes on to list at length the various forms of occupations that "fell into immediate Distress upon this Occasion," mentioning the manufacturing workers, seamstresses, milliners, cobblers, shopowners, carpenters, and so forth, who all lost their employment for want of people in the city.[31] H. F.'s own position as a "saddler" and Defoe's as the son of a butcher and tallow chandler confer even greater importance of the stalemating of such businesses.[32]

It is fairly well known that Defoe himself valued trade above all else, even morality and religious devotion.[33] Throughout his writings, Defoe evinces a "remarkable . . . consisten[cy] . . . in delineating his thoughts concerning good and bad economic practices."[34] All of this anxiety regarding the flow of international trade takes on even greater nationalistic undertones when one considers that smallpox inoculation itself was brought *to* England *from* its origins in Asia, India, and Africa. Thus, contemporary inoculation, as a medical procedure that found its origins in a foreign place and people, was a threatening import, bringing an alien practice home to London to penetrate the body of English inoculees. It is precisely for this reason that Defoe treats the hardened sores with arguably *more* anxiety than suppurated sores. Uncontrolled, leaky boundaries are anxiety-provoking for their threat to the self whose constitution rests upon an imagined separation from the other maintained by strictly defined borders. But calcified boundaries represent nothing short of paralysis, not only of British trade as a result of frozen national boundaries and trade embargoes, but also of the body itself, which will simply die if inoculative insertion of the other cannot be incorporated into the self physically and psychologically. Risk is necessary, Defoe insists again and again, through his depiction of bursting sores that connect the community and promote images of flow and ventilation. That little could be as horrifying to Defoe as the potential of stalled trade routes is nearly certain; however, when these very trade routes historically brought not only goods but also ideas and scientific methodologies such as inoculation itself, the certainty of their unhindered flow is of even more importance. Yet the borders of both trade routes and the body, when perforated, allow for the entrance of the other that is nearly as threatening. Wald's previously mentioned point that "disease emergence dramatizes the dilemma that inspires the most basic of human narratives: the necessity and danger of human contact" could not be more apt here.[35]

While the anxiety-provoking potential of perforated cutaneous sores is fairly obvious, it is the *calcified* sores of the bubonic plague that indicate just how influenced Defoe was not only by the smallpox epidemic's catalysis of inoculation, but moreover by the hobbyhorse of his economic theories that dominated so much of his life and writing. In fact, the desperate attempts to vent the fortified boundaries of an unsuppurated sore are nothing short of a synechdocal elaboration on Defoe's notions of trade generally as well as his more specific prescriptions for trade during a time of contagious epidemic.[36] For instance, a great number of critics have discussed his repeated use of the word *tokens* for the bubonic sores as having a double meaning referring to bodily sores and hearkening to currency.[37] It has already been mentioned that Defoe valued trade and commerce above nearly everything else in life. It is not surprising, then, that he states in "Of the English Trade" in his *Review:*

> The influence of trade [in England] is felt in every branch of its government . . . and the *blood* of trade is mix'd and blended with the *blood* of its gallantry, so that trade is the life of the nation . . . the spring of its wealth . . . and which (if it should sink) . . . the body politick would sicken and languish. . . . Whoever can read this, and not own with me, that to see trade sinking, declining, and in the way to ruine, ought sensibly to afflict us, must have less concern for his native country, than, I hope, all men have.[38]

Thomas Keith Meier claims that the British mercantilism of Defoe's day was characterized by a belief that the only means to the progress of the nation was through an international trade that established what the British defined as "a favourable balance of trade."[39] For the British, this "favourable" balance meant exporting more goods than it took in and importing more specie than it set forth, a "basic assertion" of British mercantilism "repeated endlessly in bullionist literature."[40] To this end, Defoe spent his career "inveigh[ing] against the belief that England could live in isolation from the other countries of Europe or the world."[41] Given the importance of international trade to him, then, "isolationist xenophobia had no attraction for Defoe."[42] Even the Dutch, ever the rivals of the British in their trading endeavors during this period, were no foe to Defoe. "No one," Bram Dijkstra notes, "was more acutely aware of the merits of Dutch methods of capital management, and of the necessity of their adoption by the English, than Defoe, who prided himself on having been . . . the Dutch-born king's personal assistant."[43] Clearly, Defoe's interests in economics had a nationalistic motivation. However, it is important to note the manner in which, even in his obvious nationalistic sentiments upholding the "nation," its "kings," and "the whole fabric" of the land, Defoe importantly addresses the relevance of trade to the "people," its individual "branch[es]," and thereby indicates the *individuals* that make up the body politic, as well as the monarch that represents it.[44]

These sentiments in "Of the English Trade" thusly illustrate not only Defoe's well-acknowledged emphasis on trade, but also his *individualistic* mercantilism. Paradoxically, while it served to support the nation at large, Defoe also depicted trade as a highly individualistic enterprise, excusing its perpetuators from the normal realm of morality and concern for others since their very trade supposedly required them to pursue their own selfish interests in order to serve national interests. Proper trade necessitated immoral, or at least amoral, acts:

> If no man must go beyond, or defraud his neighbor; if our conversation must be without covetousness, and the like, why then it is impossible for Tradesmen to be Christians, and we must unhinge all business, act upon new principles in trade, and go by new rules: in short we must shut up shop and leave off trade, and so in many things we must leave off living.[45]

In speaking of the merchant's dealings with other men, Defoe moreover claimed that "'tis *their* business to understand *him,* not his to understand them; and if he finds they do not understand him, he *will not* fail to make their ignorance to his advantage."[46] Not only did Defoe believe trade to be more important than either religion or morality, but he also in many cases indicated that proper morality and effective trade are mutually exclusive realms, given trade's emphasis on individualistic profit. Defoe nevertheless believed that the fruits of these collective individual efforts would lead to the betterment of the nation. So long as this favorable balance of trade was maintained, trade served the individual citizens of the country as well as the nation at large by "increas[ing] circulation, buying power, and the general standard of living, thereby turning the circular dance of inland trade into an ever-further soaring spiral."[47] To this end, while positing the worlds of morality and trade as necessarily parallel, he understood that private ends affected national goals, highlighting the complicated interaction of private and national spheres.

Dijkstra's use of the word *circulation* in describing eighteenth-century mercantilism is key to understanding Defoe's approval of mediated boundaries, cutaneous and otherwise. In fact, discussions of economic theory and the advantages of trade during this period relied heavily on the notion of circulation, as seen in Defoe's own aforementioned discussion of trade as that which makes the "blood of [the] gallantry" continue to flow. In 1698, Sir Charles Davenant, another political and economic commentator, described the relationship as such:[48]

> He who looks into anatomy, will wonder how life can be at all carried on, when, there are so many pipes and conduits, of which any stoppage is immediate death, and the reflection makes him melancholy. A dissection of the body politic is much of the same nature, and not at all more cheerful work.[49]

The economic theories of the seventeenth and eighteenth centuries held that such "blockages must be cleared," and asserted that it was "the task of the statesman to intervene in the circulation of wealth in order to remove impediments, to unblock pipes and conduits, to make it flow."[50] David Trotter goes so far as to assert that Defoe's heroine Roxana is not a successful businesswoman, since she is "often removed from circulation"—such is the importance of the constant flow of goods in this period, for as Trotter puts it, "a body removed from circulation accumulates rust and mold."[51] In the case of plague, rust and mold would be aptly represented rather as festering putrefaction within the garrisoned cutaneous boundaries of a calciferous bubo. Although it might seem that circulation amid the community of contagion is precisely the corporeal threat to be avoided here, Defoe's trust in trade causes him to insist rather that circulation—even amid a contagious community—is more productive than isolation; thus, he represents *instead* the calcified buboes as the stagnant force to be avoided, even at the peril of infection. As he warns in the closing words of "Of the English Trade":

[H]aving searche'd to the bottom the grievances of trade, [I] shall humbly propose what I think may remedy those evils; and then I think I have done: for my business is not to force people to accept of deliverance, but to shew them which way they may split the ship, or save it. He that will hang himself, must die.[52]

Defoe's depiction of the calcified sores and public health policy thus enacts a cyclical dynamic—it is influenced by his understanding of the significance of trade generally and, in turn, his attitude toward disease control influences his understanding of trade during times of epidemics—and the necessarily intertwined nature of trade and public welfare take on great import for him. Indeed, he closes "Of the English Trade" with a warning of jeremiadic proportions. If the reader refuses to heed his warnings about the necessity of trade circulation, he concludes, "nature can't save him, and providence will not—I shall so far act the pilot, as to place a mark upon the dangerous shoal; if the rash traders will run upon it, they must split, I can do no more."[53]

Though he clearly valued the constant circulation of international trade at all times, the unstopping of its blockages was of utmost importance during times of epidemic. To block the flow of trade normally is to stop up the arteries of the nation; to block its flow during times of contamination only allows infected sites to fester and putrefy. Of course, as aforementioned, *open* boundaries allow for the influx of the other and create, in the first place, the very potential for the inception of contamination through a risk encounter. A knee-jerk reaction to taking care of the oozing pustule might be to assume that the act of suturing its barriers back together would render it less threatening. However, it is clear that *A Journal* handles these secure cutaneous boundaries in precisely the opposite way—ripping them open and venting their contents. In this manner, Defoe illustrates that the reflex to cordon off boundaries in response to external threats is self-defeating. Rather, borders ought to be regulated and vented in a mediated manner in order to maintain circulation and prevent unmitigated seepage or even eruption.[54]

In discussing trade during the European plague outbreak of the 1720s, Defoe notes that "the main thing the Government seem to have their eyes upon in this nation is to limit and prohibit commerce with places infected, and restrain the importation of such goods as are subject to be infected."[55] While he acknowledges that the government has worked assiduously to enforce such closed borders, he qualifies his statement by observing the inefficacy of such efforts because of smugglers. Though he seems to exonerate the government here in placing the blame on individual smugglers, he importantly notes that

> [t]his vice in our commerce is introduced by the necessity this nation has been in of clogging foreign trade with heavy duties and imports, which gives encouragement to smugglers and runners of goods to venture at all hazards to bring such goods in upon us privately.[56]

Thus, Defoe underscores the fact that "clogg[ed]" trade leads to nothing more than uncontrolled and disastrous seepage. That is, in upholding trading rivalries with other countries and attempting to protect domestic trade by closing borders to potentially infected international merchandise, the British have confounded their own efforts because such fortified barriers only invite transgression. In attempting to prevent certain forms of trade before the plague, the government has done nothing short of encouraging unlawful individuals to violate these codes, a trend that persists during dangerous periods of epidemic, thus threatening the entire body politic. Although his initial statement about the aims of the government to prevent trade during periods of "distemper" seems an approbative one, it is important to keep in mind that Defoe was paid to endorse these trading quarantines and is well known for generally saying whatever he was paid to write at the moment.[57] Given his vehement disapproval of isolationist policies, however, it is unlikely that he would have truly supported such a "clogging" of the arteries of trade. Further, close examination of his language in this document reveals no actual approval of the government policy, but only an observation that their efforts "seemed sufficiently careful," which is perhaps a strategic obfuscation of his true opinion on the matter.[58] In fact, the only clear opinion he provides is simply that, had the government not "clogged" trade to begin with, it would not have had to contend with smugglers. In *A Journal*, Defoe expresses similar sentiments, though he interestingly situates infection as coming from within London and spreading outward internationally. Since "Spain and Portugal . . . would, by no means, suffer [British] Ships . . . to come into any of their ports . . . one of our Ships . . . by Stealth delivered her Cargo" there, and in this manner, "Plague was carried into these Countries by some of our Ships."[59] Here again, attempts to block trade only result in the seepage of infected trade into other nations, damaging the international trading sphere generally.

This notion, clearly rooted in his trading interests, asserts that attempts at blockades of any sort will result only in uncontrolled seepage or eruption. Such sentiments are present throughout his two longest works on the plague. Over and over again, Defoe acknowledges the threat of fully permeable boundaries during an epidemic and asserts the value therefore of the controlled perforation of borders, which allows for flow and circulation but provides some protection against infection and parasitic vitiation of the national and individual body. By allowing for the inoculative effects of mediated interactions, the individual body and the body politic may prevent complete suppuration of boundaries, thereby mitigating the enervating potential of the community of contagion. Even his seemingly ambivalent and lengthy discussion regarding the shutting up of houses, which vacillates between agreeing with the necessity of separating the sick from the well and lamenting the infringement upon human liberties, comes to rest only on the conclusion that "if the people were left at their liberty . . . those that did flee at all, would flee because [others] were infected, and thereby save their lives and likewise not carry the distemper with them when they went."[60] Thus, the shutting up of houses serves only to cause individuals— most likely infected ones—to flee in a frenzy, which spreads the contagious community's breadth to wherever they traverse. Laurel Brodsley observes that since the "language of the law disregards the community's need for social support," in its instinctive blockade against illness, the resulting confinement becomes "psychologically and spiritually onerous," resulting in breakouts and runaways that cause a total "reversal of the intended result of this policy."[61] Indeed, though H. F. considers the matter from different angles throughout the text, he comes to the conclusion that "it was rather hurtful," since (as he delineates in a typically Defoean list):

> (1st) of all, [it was] not effectual, but that the People broke out, whether by Force or by Stratagem, even almost as often as they pleas'd: And (2d) that those that did thus break out, were generally People infected, who in their Desperation, running about from one Place to another, valued not who they injur'd.[62]

Attempting to quarantine and fully blockade diseased individuals results only in infecting a greater number of them because when they are shut up in a home together through involuntary confinement, this results in an inevitable eruption of infected bodies that are likely to burst forth and infect a greater number of people. If, rather, people were left as they were, *un*infected individuals could leave infected areas as they pleased, extricating themselves from the community of contagion through permeable boundaries, thereby preventing the catastrophic eruption of the plague to all the country. Instead of fortified quarantines, Defoe again advocates a system of regulated, but permeable boundaries whereby

> [t]he sound people of the town be immediately removed and obliged to go to some certain particular place, where barracks should be built for them . . . and where they should be obliged to perform a quarantine of days, and after that to be admitted to go whither they pleased, *except* back to the town from whence they came.[63]

Thus, by cordoning off individuals from one another, but allowing them regulated access to certain areas, society may both regulate the community of contagion and prevent its stagnation and overflow.

Permeable Borders as a Mode of Survival

In addition to suggesting general public health strategies that catalyze regulated but permeable borders, Defoe makes his case about the benefits of mediated flow through extended specific examples that he sets up nearly as self-help manuals for readers' guidance. The first portion of Defoe's *Due Preparations*, for instance, consists mostly of a lengthy description of a man who represents, for Defoe, a model for defending against the plague. He sets aside stores of food for his family and quarantines them voluntarily from the rest of the population while they are still well—hearkening to Defoe's repeated insistence that voluntary sequestration is highly preferable to forced quarantines. Underscoring his emphasis on maintaining trade flow and circulation, Defoe likens the man's preparations for his family's removal to trading expeditions to "Barbadoes or Jamaica."[64] After gathering food and shutting his family up, he constructs a number of portals that allow access to his house, but mediate any such access due to their size. He shuts all his windows "except the wooden shutter kept open for conversing"[65] with necessary outsiders and hires a porter who acts as mediator for him and his family, thus further controlling even the access to the small "wicket" he constructs in his door, which serves to "take in or give out anything they thought fit."[66] Even the windows in the man's house speak to Defoe's assertion of the necessity of mediated permeability. When the man "nail[s] up all the casements of his windows," Defoe adds an editorial footnote, observing that "they had no sash windows in those days, nor for many years after."[67] Here, Defoe cleverly ropes even window design into his insistence upon mediated boundaries, hinting that sash windows (whose openings are smaller than casement windows) afford greater regulation of an area of permeation and are therefore more desirable. Defoe presents all of these mechanisms in the home as safeguards not only against the contamination threatened by completely unmediated contact with others during times of contagion, but also against the paralysis of complete isolation, which serves only to clog and stagnate the individual and the national body.[68]

Empathetic Connection as a Prerequisite to Survival in Mary Shelley's *The Last Man*

Though I would stretch his argument back to the Enlightenment period of Defoe, Fuson Wang is quite correct in noting the Romantic period's emphasis "on a porous disease discourse" (468). In the time between *A Journal of the Plague Year* and *The Last Man*, William Jenner's work had shifted practice from variolation to vaccination. The riskier procedure of inoculation with virulent smallpox material gave way to inoculation with the relatively harmless cowpox (the procedure renamed "vaccination" after the Latin word for "cow"). In the process, vaccination thus became more widespread in practice, and also carried with it a more mediated sense of risk to the general public, who were increasingly compelled to comply with the procedure. While both Defoe's and Shelley's texts occur before bacteriology and germ theory would take the world by storm, both are marked by the imagery of the inoculation/ vaccine techne of their time. One hundred years apart though these texts are, they stand as helpful signposts indicating authorial resistance to neoliberal bioethics of isolation and self-preservation. In fact, this chronological gap makes visible the impact of socioscientific discourse on risk assessment and risk aversion. Yoked by common concerns, Mary Shelley takes up a similar argument to Defoe's in *The Last Man* (1826), in which she similarly insists on permeability and the value of risk encounters—often via depiction of the stultifying effects of isolationist impulses. Here, the very nature of England's island topography is initially perceived as a protective force against the tide of contagion. This topographically grounded isolationist impulse is little more than a false sense of security, however, as Britain is ultimately enveloped in the epidemic by others seeking the theoretical safety of its insular situation. The power of Shelley's imaginative construction lies in her simultaneous display of the universal human imperative toward self-preservation alongside her demonstration of the futility and self-defeating nature of such aims. *The Last Man* thusly sympathizes with these fruitless human impulses while it concomitantly promotes sympathetic encounters with the other.

Shelley's bioethical admonitions begin broadly, tracing what she casts as the natural human tendency toward self-protective instincts, seen initially in the characters' belief that their isolation on an island will protect them; she then demonstrates that in an increasingly globalized society, not only is there no such possibility of true quarantine, but also, much as Defoe demonstrated before her, such attempts at quarantine only lead to panicked overflow of infection. Alan Bewell calls this imperative "the imaginative center of [Shelley's] novel."[69] Humans exist "on an earth unified by the continual movement of people, goods, and pathogens."[70] As such, "there are no safe places, and nobody is exempt from possible contact."[71] There are no class- or nation-based boundaries against contagion, since (as Defoe and Shelley recognized more poignantly perhaps because of their pre-germ-theory epistemological frameworks) as humans are inextricably "entangled . . . in the web of society," "the atmosphere . . . as a cloak enwraps all our fellow creatures" together within this web, in "every nook of our spacious globe."[72] The influence of Defoe's ethical imperatives as a model for Shelley's own is explicitly stated numerous times in the novel—the narrator, Verney, repeatedly alludes to him and his *Journal of the Plague Year* by name. When the plague first appears in London, Verney recounts that many citizens looked to *A Journal of the Plague Year* to divine the future and, perhaps, gain wisdom from narrator H. F.'s strategies.[73] Shelley's Romantic text thus acts as an apt conceptual bridge between Defoe's early osmotic ideals and the later isolationist and antiseptic impulses that became prevalent in society after the 1860s. *The Last Man* moves from Defoe's heavily mercantile value on openness to more patently bioethical arguments for connection, compassion, and mediated risk encounters in a world that had become more saturated with epidemiological techne. In so doing, Shelley builds upon his early inoculation-informed politics and also foregrounds the anti-isolationist moves of the late-century authors covered in the rest of this book.

Writing just after the revolutionary fervor of the late eighteenth century, and being grounded in the Romantic tradition as she is, Shelley also incorporates a great deal of discussion of the body politic under pressure in *The Last Man*. In fact, nearly the first half of the novel has very little to do with plague at all, and is largely comprised of one family's involvement with a politically powerful family in a future Britain (the year is 2021) transitioning from a monarchy to a republic. All of these factors lend to Shelley's alignment with Defoe in her insistence on the value of open global trade. At first glance, this consumerist motivation is surprising to see in Shelley's work, more so than in Defoe's, for whom such mercantile sentiments are predictably ubiquitous. However, her use of this topic reveals itself to be much more about community (rather than commerce) than it first appears. Like Defoe, Shelley highlights the near-universal drive toward self-preservation via quarantine and, of course, simultaneously demonstrates the futility of these efforts as guaranteed by the very form of an apocalyptic story. "Nations," Verney recounts, "bordering on the already infected countries, began to enter upon serious plans for the better keeping out of the enemy."[74] Verney recounts Britain's response to such global moves as paradoxical; he juxtaposes the global response with Britain's reliance on trade for survival, which at once heightens the threat of both quarantine and open trade: "We, a commercial people, were obliged to bring such schemes under consideration."[75] However, the inscrutability of the plague's mode of communication gives the British "legislators pause before they could decide on the laws to be put in force."[76] Thus, even while Verney acknowledges that "no prevention could be judged superfluous, which even added a chance to [Britain's] escape" from contamination, nevertheless, Verney embeds into his discussion of government legislation the idea that national and trade quarantines are ineffective at best.[77] His assessment of the dilemma emphasizes a moderate, osmotic approach, evenhandedly recognizing that "the cost of maintaining Britain as a social environment prevents it from isolating itself from the rest of the world" fully.[78] However, as an apocalyptic novel, Shelley takes the question of trade embargoes to its logical conclusion. Even though Britain eventually opts to keep ports open, trade is unavoidably "palsied" as the global population dies off and there is nobody left to trade with.[79] In discussing the collapse of global trade, Shelley draws upon the circulatory imagery so fundamental to Defoe's discussion of economics during times of crisis. In spite of England's desire to continue trade and maintain permeable borders, "the great heart of mighty Britain was pulseless. Commerce had ceased."[80] Thus, in intensifying the tenor of the dilemma from Defoe's tone of political lobbying to one of helpless acceptance (Britain in fact can no longer *choose* to engage in trade) Shelley deftly shores up her argument and demonstrates—via absence—the vitalizing properties of community, both global and local.

While continuing Defoe's trend of insisting that effective quarantine is neither possible nor helpful, Shelley foregrounds the reactions of the later authors I cover in the remainder of this book by insisting additionally that such self-protective isolation reduces humanity to *zoē*, or bare life. As Shelley puts it, such efforts "ben[d] the highest objects of human ambition" and "converge them to one point"—pure survival.[81] It is important to note, of course, the paradoxical fact that Verney spends portions of the book going to great lengths to find a place to take his family that is safe from the disease. However, the main characters' search for "uncontaminated seclusion" predominantly takes the form of mediated contact, as seen in the small, manageable communities the group forms in various locations, where the sick and the well dwell together. It is also worth noting here that in spite of their eventual efforts at self-preservation via isolation, the group stays engaged with and active in the community until the population of England has dwindled to such an extent that it is impossible to continue to build upon community there; only then do they determine to seek others outside of the island's bounds. Thus, what can look like the protagonist's pursuit of isolation and self-preservation are actually moves that remain rooted in and motivated by community. Bioethics aside, Shelley and Defoe's messages about the impossibility of effective quarantine also remain one and the same, since Verney is entirely unsuccessful in protecting his family from death (through various forms of infection and drowning). Although the group clings to the dwindling community they have remaining in the last portion of the book, they grow to realize they are inhabiting *zoē*, in negative correlation with the declining local population of their traveling group. "To live," Verney says in growing awareness of this fact, "we must not only observe and learn, we must also feel; we must not be mere spectators of action, we must act."[82] Increasingly, Shelley builds into Verney's story images of risk encounters—symbolic inoculative gestures—which indicate that some exposure to risk is not only inevitable but potentially vitalizing.

Defoe's osmotic bioethics emerged from his direct encounter of the 1721 smallpox outbreak and the subsequent experimentation with inoculation. Shelley, so parallel in her aims to Defoe, also lived through a smallpox epidemic in 1816. Importantly, this was the first smallpox outbreak in Britain subsequent to Jenner's adaptation of vaccination procedures from the Eastern techne of inoculation brought to England by Mary Wortley Montague in Defoe's era.[83] Because inoculation involved incorporating actual smallpox pathogens into the body, whereas vaccination drew upon the protection imparted by the non-lethal cowpox, debates raged fiercely after the 1816 epidemic about which method was most advisable—that is, just how much of a risk encounter with the diseased other should one hazard in seeking to preserve life. William Woodville most famously rejected the notion that vaccination provided as much immunity from smallpox as inoculation, arguing that logic dictated that "the advantages to be derived from substituting the cow-pox for the small-pox must be directly in proportion to the greater mildness of the former."[84] As history reflects, of course, Jenner was victorious in the promotion of vaccination. He was not without continued opposition, however, as our present-day anti-vaxx movement indicates.

Shelley's novel resists such discussions about incorporating the least possible risk necessary, and instead embraces—often quite literally—the risky other as exemplary of a meaningful life. During a military skirmish about halfway through the plot, Adrian halts the opposing troops, urging them not to "be more pitiless than pestilence," and to not only refrain from violent acts, but even to embrace the potentially diseased bodies of those around them. To add pathos to his speech, he cradles a bleeding body, from which "the warm tide of life gushed" while he speaks.[85] Here, while Adrian discusses the evils of military violence, he simultaneously physically embraces the risk of blood-borne pathogens carrying plague, while "every heart, late . . . bent on universal massacre, now beat anxiously in hope . . . [for] this one sufferer."[86] This intimate encounter vividly highlights the paradox that pursuit of the bare life frequently results in neglect of the meaningful minutiae that make life worth pursuing. The soldiers fighting over the remaining scraps of resources left in England pursue biological life with ferocity, are moved by Adrian's risky acceptance of the bloody other into his arms, and begin to see "the fate of the world . . . bound up in the death of this single man."[87]

The inoculative risk encounters in *The Last Man* do not stop at simple encounters with the other, but proceed to depictions of literal inoculative immunity. Adrian, for one, is read by some critics to be somehow immune to the plague, although his explanation suggesting this interpretation is vague and the accuracy of his assumption—for assumption it remains throughout the book—is questionable.[88] When Verney resists Adrian's determination to stay in the community and help the remaining survivors, Adrian responds matter-of-factly: "as to my peculiar liability to infection, I could easily prove, both logically and physically, that in the midst of contagion I have a better chance of life than you."[89] While some have read this as Adrian's immunity, I would point out that Adrian does not use the word *plague*, which is used as a rule throughout the novel to refer to the specific infection at hand. I suggest, rather, that this bold proclamation expresses a Romantic sense of individual differences in constitutional susceptibility to infection, rather than a specific immunity. The context of their discussion, to my thinking, supersedes debate about the precise meaning of his statement here. In this scene, Adrian is arguing with Verney about his resolution to stay among his community members and aid them during the plague. As I will return to later, his use of "life" here takes on implications beyond the suggestion of biological viability, when his statement is understood to indicate his openness to risk and service-oriented community involvement.

Another example will serve to make this point clearer. A woman named Martha appears in an isolated episode; she is also clearly inoculated, and the mode of such protection is here explicit: she contracted the plague but recovered, and is thereafter immune to its effects. She, like Adrian, refuses to stay isolated in self-satisfied immunity, but brings food and supplies to the community and "shew[s] them how the well-being of each include[s] the prosperity of all."[90] The most famous inoculative moment in the novel, of course—although deeming it such has itself been the subject of much critical debate[91]—is Verney's own encounter with an infectious individual who reaches out and clutches him:

> I felt my leg clasped, and a groan repeated by the person that held me. I . . . saw a negro half-clad, writhing under the agony of disease, while he held me with a compulsive grasp. With mixed horror and impatience I strove to disengage myself, and fell on the sufferer; he wound his naked festering arms around me, his face was so close to mine, and his breath, death-laden, entered my vitals.[92]

More critical debate focuses on this one moment than perhaps any other in the novel. Interpretations are polarized. Some view this scene as a consciously penned embrace of the other, a willingness to encounter risk (particularly as this encounter is here racialized). Conversely, given that Verney is overcome with "horror" and subsequently "thr[ows] the wretch from [him]" in disgust, some critics argue that this is a clear moment of absolute aversion to an unwanted encounter, and signals little more than racialized othering of the plague itself, a thinly veiled stand-in for the self-congratulatory voice of British superiority.[93] It is beyond the scope of the present project to outline the colonial endeavors that informed and were informed by scientific concepts of cell biology and germ theory; Laura Otis and Alan Bewell have done so in their powerful books, which address this subject at great length. There are inarguably important racial and political dynamics to issues of biomedicine, and rather than gloss over them reductively here, I direct the reader to these important texts. For the purposes of my own argument here—images of mediated risk encounters subsequent to the development of variolation (in Defoe) and vaccination (in Shelley)—suffice it to say that regardless of how one reads this scene, most critics agree that this encounter provides Verney his immunity and enables his survival and the survival of *The Last Man* as a textual artifact. Averse though he may be to his risk encounter—and Shelley heightens his sense of being "othered" through the vehicle of racial embodiment—it nevertheless occurs and provides the immunity that makes Shelley's message possible. Through this episode, then, Shelley underscores the urgency of her ethical imperative: (1) disease does not recognize socially constructed barriers of race, class, gender, or nation; (2) therefore, humans cannot avoid disease, try as they might; and (3) were they willing to engage with some amount of risk rather than indulging in futile efforts at self-preservation and isolation, they would find that the effort expands the scope of life beyond the biological and into the fulfilling and meaningful. They might, as with Adrian, "in the midst of contagion . . . have a better chance of *life*."[94]

To take this point even farther, Shelley also depicts a series of proto-an-ti-vaxxers, as it were, into her novel, demonstrating the enervating impact of such contact-averse strategies. Like Defoe's anecdote about a woman who is so horrified by the buboes on her daughter's body that she goes mad on the spot, running away from her own child, Shelley, too, describes a mother who shuns even her own children. Foregrounding the concerns of the late Victorian period, Shelley alters the Defoean setup only slightly such that the woman is avoiding all human contact *prophylactically*, not just those who are visibly already diseased. The woman, though more than one hundred years old, is determined that the plague will not take her, and "cling[s] . . . to the remnant of her spent life," which is here clearly demarcated by this narrative editorializing as the bare life, particularly insofar as the woman excommunicates herself from society the moment she hears someone in her local community has the plague.[95] From that moment, she "barred her door, and closed her casement, refusing to communicate with any."[96] Unlike Defoe's rather inventive suggestion of casement windows as osmotic media-tors, the woman in Shelley's example enacts a total *cordon sanitaire*. Initially, her son, who is not exempt from her principle of isolation, "humor[s] her by placing articles of food" near her home.[97] After he dies of the plague, the woman must forage for her own food. She does so at night, judging that she is likely to meet fewer people, and every day returns home, under increasing threat of starvation, merely "pleased that she [had] met no one," here a metonym for the self-assurance that "she was in no danger from the plague."[98] In spite of her increasing difficulty in procuring food, "her greatest care [is] to avoid her fellow creatures," come what may.[99] What comes, is, of course, plague. Reposing one night during a bout of weakness while foraging, she hears the cries of a dying plague victim begging for water. Predictably, she ignores the sufferer, whose contamination she has so long dreaded, but she is forcibly confronted with the victim's presence, when he or she (the individual's sex is never mentioned) grabs her hand, crying out with relief and joy at having found another human presence to relieve his/her dying moments. "At last you are come!" the sufferer cries, before dying, all the while clinging to the woman's arm. The woman is horrified by the failure of all her careful planning. Instantly, she "believe[s] herself to be infected," and so "no longer dread[s] the association of others; but, as swiftly as she might, comes to her grand-daughter, at Windsor Castle, there to lament and die."[100] The point of this microcosm of a case study is that this woman was not only alone for her last months, but opted out of her son's dying moments, as well, only to be confronted in the end with the unavoidable physical (and, by implication, social and moral) connection to others around her. One would hesitate to say the woman has changed or grown by the time of her death, as her impulses seem purely self-serving to the end. However, in this episode, buried as it is in the midst of the larger narrative of England's decline and depopulation, Shelley turns a mirror onto the reader, illuminating what she depicts as a universal drive toward self-preservation, and her isolationist anecdotes drive home her "critique [of] scientific generalizations that ignore the fate of individuals."[101] One hears the somewhat cutting ring of the golden rule at the episode's conclusion, as the woman herself refuses to be alone in her dying moments, and seems unconcerned with her contaminating potential unto others. Intriguingly, the old woman's anecdote and another more general reference to "instances of desertion and even murders" in the hopes of escaping contagion occasion the peculiar use of the word *dastard* in the text.[102] The general deserters, who hope to "be among the elect" survivors "cl[i]ng to life with dastard tenacity," while the elderly woman is said to "cling" with a "dastard feeling" to life.[103] Although colloquially "dastard" has become a somewhat archaic term for the mustache-twirling villains of yore, the word actually specifically refers to the mediated risk encounters Defoe and Shelley advocate. The *OED* cites the word as meaning "one who meanly or basely shrinks from danger . . . so as not to expose himself to risk." Ad hominem judgments of cowardice aside, the episodic anecdotes in the novel clearly indicate that such efforts to avoid risk exposure are futile to begin with, as disease does not obey social and national boundaries, and are liable only to reduce the quality of communal life or result in eruptive violence. Moreover, in the post-Jenner world of vaccination that Shelley was writing from, her admonitions about the vitalizing value of risk encounters and her depictions of inoculative contact engage one another in a socioscientific discursive cycle. In a world increasingly globalized and formed to serve colonial endeavors, Shelley "insist[s] that Western societies cannot isolate themselves from the world they have helped create."[104] As Verney himself says in addressing a small crowd of Londoners, "our risk is common; our precautions and exertions shall be common also."[105]

Disease states rawly expose these animalistic instincts, so to speak, toward self-preservation, and Shelley demonstrates here that no one is immune from the innate drive to live, when and if the drive to *thrive* has become impossible. In the same speech to the public, Shelley demonstrates that even Verney is not free from this universal hope for biological survival, as he boldly proclaims that "plague will not find [England] a ready prey. We will dispute every inch of ground; and, by methodical and inflexible laws, pile invincible barriers to the progress of our foe."[106] A desire to be "among the elect" survivors, as Verney has earlier put it, is of course universal—and this will especially play into the antiseptic fantasies and isolationist drives of the post-germ-theory world covered in the following chapters. Shelley's awareness of this is evident, and hence, like Defoe, she advocates moderation and openness, not simple bravado or martyrdom. Shelley is keenly aware that disease is an apt vehicle for explicating these notions, as disease strips us of our speciesist certainty that we are automatically endowed with a life that is somehow more than the sum of our cellular parts—that we can live, that is, more than the bare life.

The Last Man works as a jeremiad, then, warning against the consequences of the division and perpetuation of biological life maintained at the expense of emotional meaning or spiritual fulfillment. If an apocalyptic novel is successful, it will warn readers *away* from the actions depicted in the story, and will thusly turn out *not* to be "true" in terms of future events. Shelley taps into this potential throughout the book, particularly with anecdotes of contagion avoided and nevertheless contracted. Efforts at complete aseptic isolation are not only futile but harmful, and they are moreover shortsighted. Whether imbued in the "pernicious effluvia" of certain locales as miasma once contended, or transmitted via "deathly exhalations" as germ theory would later posit, contamination indeed pervades the "atmosphere which enwraps all our fellow creatures."[107] We simply cannot avoid its reach. In attempting to do so, we only reduce the span of our necessarily limited existence to a protracted circle of pure biological life. There has, in fact, been much critical debate about the epidemiological nature of the plague in *The Last Man,* largely because Shelley vacillates between miasmatic and contagious discursive practices in describing it.[108] As well versed as Shelley clearly is in both sides of this epistemological model, however, I would argue that critics miss the point with readings that attempt to hem in her amorphous pathogen. Both her personal background and her informed use of both miasmatic discourse and contagion rhetoric indicate a conscious representational ambiguity.[109] For Shelley, the precise mode of contagion is less important than the social experiment she plays out before the reader's eyes. If the story of the empty last days of the elderly woman was not clear enough for readers, Shelley incorporates a bleaker specter into the novel in the form of none other than the Black Spectre. After the company has left England and set out for the Continent, gaining a few more party members as they travel, the group begins to witness a "Black Spectre" on the edges of their campsite each night. At first, the group sees in this figure the image of death, looming in their future, until they coincidentally stumble upon the figure itself, dead in the road. Verney explains that the ominous Black Spectre was merely a "French noble" who was the lone survivor in his community. In his solitude, he

> had wandered from town to town, from province to province, seeking some survivor for a companion, and abhorring the loneliness to which he was condemned. When he discovered our troop, fear of contagion conquered his love of society. He dared not join us, yet he could not resolve to lose sight of us, sole human beings who besides himself existed in . . . France.[110]

If the image of the reclusive mother were not sufficient to drive home Shelley's point, she reiterates the notion with the Black Spectre, who is always referred to by this eponym of allegorical proportions. Robbed of all community, the man is desperate to maintain visual contact with Verney's traveling party. Fearful of contagion, however, he only pursues the connection this far. Thus, he hovers on the outskirts of the group, so desperate for and yet fearful of connection. But in keeping his distance, he maintains only the imaginative potential of this community until his death, alone on the road. Although the group has superstitiously interpreted his figure as the "Black Spectre" of Death looming in their future, when the group later stumbles across his unconscious body in the road and learns of his story just before his death, Shelley in fact reveals the "Black Spectre" to be the bleak rewards of pursuit of bare life. Death is, of course, an inevitable outcome of biological life; this is writ large in the imaginative scenario of apocalyptic plague in *The Last Man*. Shelley's project across the length of *The Last Man*, then, uses the apocalyptic form to warn not against plague and disease so much as the potential for society to buy into neoliberal ideology by pursuing and even valorizing the bare life—here represented as biological survival *in vacuo*. If Adrian's ability to maintain "life amidst contagion" is a life of meaning rather than of biology, then the Black Spectre's death is a shadow of the community life he avoided, rather than the biological life from which he departed.[111]

This growing awareness is most fully articulated in Verney's horror in the last portion of the book at being, in fact, the eponymous last man. Just before he is quite the very last man, however, he laments the dwindling numbers of his companions:

> [W]e alone—we three—alone—alone—sole dwellers on the sea and on the earth, we three must perish! The vast universe, its myriad worlds, and the plains of boundless earth which we had left—the extent of shoreless sea around—contracted to my view—they and all that they contained, shrunk up to one point, even to our tossing bark, freighted with glorious humanity.[112]

As his entourage diminishes in number, the group increasingly seeks out paintings and artistry as a desperate means of communing with others via their expressive artifacts. Finally, when he is assured that he is indeed the "last man," Verney even begins to read again. He and his companions have hitherto generally avoided reading, because it too vividly recalled human life that no longer signified for the lone survivors. This, of course, is a thinly veiled commentary on Shelley's part about the power of her medium of choice to communicate important truths about human connections. Paradoxically, "as the lonely state of singleness" further "hems [him] in," Verney travels to Rome and contemplates prose.[113] He meditates upon this renewed source of connection with other humans: "the verses of Horace and Virgil . . . thronged into the opened gates of my mind, [and] I felt myself exalted by the long forgotten enthusiasm."[114] His renewed ability to find a source of connection to other people, even across the threshold of bare life and mortality, leads to an actualized and fulfilled *existence* for Verney. He excitedly recounts:

> I was delighted to know that I beheld the scene which they beheld—the scene which their wives and mothers and crowds of the unnamed witnessed, while at the same time they honoured, applauded, or wept for these matchless specimens of humanity.[115]

After plague has made it clear that nationalistic and class-based pretensions are inept means of stabilizing self-protective notions (whether of superiority or simple, bare life), Verney proceeds to the book's conclusion with the surprisingly egalitarian notion that each and every life is "matchless" in its provision of meaningful points of connection and communion with the social realm deemed so threatening in times of contagious crisis. Now, having achieved the status of the "elect" survivor, he realizes this for the hollow victory that it is, exclaiming, "Without love, without sympathy, without communion with any, how could I meet the morning sun?"[116] Reconnected to vicarious human connection through artistic artifacts, Verney movingly concludes that this human connection is the *only* cure for inscrutable catastrophe. He "had found a consolation" for despair in even this distanced form of human connection. That is, he elaborates, he "had discovered a medicine for [his] many and vital wounds," and that medicine is none other than a disavowal of the instinct toward self-preservation at the expense of community encounters.[117]

Narrator-Survivors: Embedding Life in Death

Embedded in the narrative voice of both novels is this very dilemma: the very nature of apocalyptic plague fiction implies the existence of a narrator-survivor left to tell the story. In these novels, Defoe and Shelley insist on textual veracity via "live-time" statistical updates and prefatory material, respectively. The existence of the supposedly nonfictional texts themselves additionally implies the existence of a continued audience within the imagined community of the story. Shelley's narrator literally incorporates her admonitions about the pursuit of a meaningful life within community over the preservation of bare, biological life. Thus, Verney's own striving for community and meaningful communication is first sought in his own reading, and then in his reaching outward toward a readership.

Defoe's narrator, H. F., likewise embodies Defoe's insistence on osmotic openness as a public health and private existential method of preservation. While Verney must necessarily have died long before the excavation of his manuscript by a much later, nameless preface-writer, H. F.'s corpse is *incorporated* into his own narrative, thereby rendering his own body—present and absent, survivor and victim, narrator and narrated—permeable. H. F. defies the supposedly insuperable boundaries of text and non-text as he tiptoes along the borders of his own narrative, telling his story in the face of an anonymously appended editorial note that informs his readership of his death in a mass plague burial pit in London. Wafting in and out of his own text, then, a ghostly shade of the supposedly immune epidemiologist that *was* historically and *is* textually, H. F. permeates even the boundaries of his own text and livelihood. In his liminal existence, he acts as Defoe's finest exemplar of permeable boundaries and their healthy effect upon circulatory systems of all sorts, as it is his narration that allows the text itself to circulate, eventually finding itself in the hands of the reader.[118] Every element of Defoe's most extensive plague texts serves to underscore his insistence on mediated boundaries that allow for circulation of goods and people; this very fact further emphasizes his notion that every individual body maintained through mediated permeability within this system serves the greater good of facilitating national trade circulation—and therefore regulated national osmosis—in the aggregate.

This insistence on openness to risk encounters is taken up by Shelley's narrator, who has acknowledged H. F.'s influence on his strategies and understanding of plague. At the conclusion of his manuscript, he further urges the importance of community, if life is to extend beyond purely neoliberal bounds. He does so, like H. F., through the synthesis of the verisimilitude of his text and his own liminal posthumous voice captured therein. He leaves his text, he laments, "for whom to read?—to whom dedicated?" His question breaks the fourth wall, forcing readers to attend to their own vitality, since they are, of course, alive and reading the book Verney is actively insisting none will read. In the very next lines, Verney pushes his ostensibly rhetorical question to its logical conclusion and dedicates his book to "the illustrious dead," "shadows" whom he commands: "arise and read your fall."[119] If apocalyptic narratives are only as successful as they are inaccurate prophecies, Shelley adds further chronological layers to her novel in order to ensure its efficacy vis-à-vis inaccuracy: Verney's manuscript is supposedly constructed by an anonymous editor, who found the text in a Sibylline cave in 1818. Verney's manuscript, while dated as occurring in 2021, are in fact ancient prophecies (the Sibyl being an ancient Greek oracle of sorts). Thus, Shelley allows for her futuristic vision to remain a mere possibility, a fate that can still be avoided by audiences in 1818 who can alter the string of future events and possibly find themselves facing a different fate in 2021, when it finally arrives. This chronological vacillation heightens the jeremiadic heft of the novel's warning, and also adds to the permeable boundaries that Verney, like H. F. before him (and whom he has somehow read in his prophetic vision from Ancient Greece), treads.

Having at this point been schooled by Verney in the fates of the elderly woman and, more heavy-handedly, that of the Black Spectre, whose death was an existential death during life, living readers who necessarily exist in a state of biological life in order to engage with Verney's manuscript (and, by proxy, Shelley's book) are in fact the ones addressed by his dedication. When Verney commands his readers, therefore, to "arise, and read your fall," it is a spiritual death of the bare neoliberal life that Verney portends as the true "fall" of his apocalyptic manuscript. Performing her role as supposed editor, Shelley, then, indeed encourages her audience to "arise" and "read," lest they become "shadows" like Verney's Black Spectre and not only complacently accept, but in fact pursue a bare life which constitutes the "nucleus of sovereign power."[120] This, too, functions as an osmotic gesture in its liminal existence, and simultaneously as an invitation to engage in inoculative activities, by insisting on the persisting value of human encounters, risky though they necessarily are. The narrative frame "re-present[s] the narrator's mediated version of the story, insisting that this tale of a dead-end history be opened back up to reader responsiveness, back to that most important of human feelings, sympathy."[121]

Nancy Armstrong and Leonard Tennenhouse have noted Defoe's ability to envision a form of the body politic that allows for the mass of the body ruled by a sovereign, but also takes into account and allows for the possibility of the individuation of each of the constitutive people within the body politic itself. In so doing, Defoe holds in tension the notion of an unindividuated mass of people who give over their rights to the sovereign and the necessarily individuated actions of the people that make up this body. In his unique view of the body politic, Defoe "found the concept of the individual ineffective as an antidote to contagion."[122] That is, in a community of contagion, no individual effort can succeed at limiting the collective force of infection that circulates through the entire body of the people. Instead, Defoe illustrates a world in which "the very circulation spreading the plague begins to limit, check, and finally nullify it."[123] In this world, which has "neither a sovereign nor sovereign individuals," the health of the individual-as-self and individual-as-national-subject is "limited only by the extent of its flow and the supply of goods and information . . . [and it] thrives most when all its parts are healthy, just as the whole deteriorates when any part is visited by the plague."[124] Thus, the circulatory capacity of the people trapped within a plague-afflicted community is the only defense against the paralytic forces of the contagious community itself. Likewise, Shelley's temporal distortion and framing techniques in her novel "trust in the moral possibilities" of humanity's "imaginative capability for sympathy and its enlightened capability for community," which she suggests is recoverable "so long as sympathetic exchange between two persons, modeled by the relationship of the frame narrator to reader, actor to audience, remains possible."[125]

This solution, which separates portions of its solute out while it holds them in stasis within a seemingly contradictory solvent, is typical of Defoe's treatment of the plague in *A Journal.* Over and over in this plague treatise, he insists: closed boundaries stagnate; open borders allow for life-giving circulation. While he certainly reacts to the virulent potential of suppurated cutaneous boundaries that threaten to rob the individual and national body of selfhood, he also resists the instinct to revolt against such horrors by simply closing off these boundaries. Instead of presenting calciferous sores as a safe haven, then, Defoe depicts these seemingly safeguarded sites of infection rather as more contagious effusions, simply waiting to erupt if their contents are not safely vented. In response to this understanding, Defoe—likely influenced by the smallpox outbreak in London just before he penned *A Journal*—advocates for an inoculative gesture both in trade (in order to maintain the body politic) and in personal living (in order to maintain the individual subjectivities that form that body). Clogging, stagnation, and noxious overflow can only be avoided by resisting the self-preserving impulse to cordon off the self or the other completely and instead allowing for a bit of the other to be taken into the self in a controlled manner. These mediations of flow across borders prevent the eventual eruption of closed boundaries and allow for the healthy circulation of the individual and the national body. Defoe's openness to the mysterious other—his cautious willingness to probe and penetrate the imaginary membranes that seem to keep us safe from unwanted intruders—ultimately invites readers to adopt a humanitarian sense of openness and contact in a globalizing world where the necessary reliance of English subjects on foreign bodies is increasingly hard to ignore. As Shelley would later put it, drawing upon and expanding Defoe's communalism to an even broader openness toward encounters with risk that move humanity beyond the bare life, "let us leave 'life,' that we may live."[126]

"A Speculative Idea"

Childbed Fever, Early Germ Theory Debates, and (En)Gendered Speculation in Henry James's *Washington Square*

The physician must do something. He cannot remain a spectator merely.

—Walter Channing, *A Treatise on Etherization in Childbirth: Illustrated by Five Hundred and Eighty-One Cases*

The doctor enjoyed the point he had made. It came to Catherine with the force—or rather with the vague impressiveness—of a logical axiom which it was not in her province to controvert; and yet, though it was a scientific truth, she felt wholly unable to accept it.

—Henry James, *Washington Square*

Radical Isolation: Subverting a Subversion

Leaving "life" in order "to live" took many forms in later Victorian literature, as the following chapters will show. Henry James's *Washington Square* exemplifies the same emphasis on community explored in the last chapter, but accomplishes this paradoxically through a prolonged consideration of one woman's lifelong isolation. In so doing, this novel is an apt illustration of the manner in which late-Victorian authors often held risk and community in tension with one another in their literature. Beginning with James, we can see in the literature of this era a refusal to depict human interaction as simplistic or easily reducible to utilitarian terms of "good" or "bad." Rather, many authors pushed back against the isolationist ideologies of quarantine-based purity, but they did not do this through reductive or maudlin portrayals of martyrdom. Their works do not invite purposeful contraction of disease and encounters with death, but rather insist that risk, and particularly risk from contact with other bodies and minds, is intricately tied up with life; to avoid it, or rather to engage in the futile attempt to do so, can only mean death of the self in a way perhaps more significant than physical un-being.

Washington Square is in many ways a typically Jamesian novella—light on plot and heavy on character development. Catherine Sloper is an heiress in the first half of the nineteenth century whose father, a "ladies' doctor,"[2] refuses to authorize her marriage to Morris Townsend, a probable fortune hunter with whom she has fallen in love. Seemingly anticlimactically, the novel ends with Catherine both refusing to promise her father that she will never marry Morris (thereby exempting herself from his will), but also choosing never to marry him. She remains single in her father's house for the rest of her life. It may seem counterintuitive to include a novel about a protagonist who ends her life in solitude as part of a study of authorial insistence upon community. However, the plot of *Washington Square* paradoxically upholds the value of community when the text is read in light of the fact that the novel and its characters are explicitly situated within the context of early germ theory debates and the gendered arena of obstetrical science in which they were fought.

Like Shelley, James employs temporal dissonances in *Washington Square*: the novel was written at the height of germ theory's popularity and widespread acceptance in the 1880s, but the story is *set* in germ theory's infancy, the 1840s. In this earlier period, the seemingly uncorrelated trajectories of gender biases, germ theory, and obstetrical science in fact coalesced in a mutually constitutive path of disastrous risky encounters and, consequentially, the development of changed cultural attitudes toward risk and willingness to encounter the other. While Shelley's apocalyptic novel uses temporal distortion to set up a warning for a society unwilling to listen to the moral of her story, James uses temporal distancing to exert external control as to exactly what moral readers discern at the story's conclusion.

Washington Square is therefore a prime example of the necessity of meaningfully tying literature to its contemporary scientific contexts and, perhaps more importantly, of contextualizing that science within the culture that produced it.[3] Through temporal prestidigitation, James focuses audience attention on a specific set of external contexts, and the somewhat plodding, uneventful plot of the novel metamorphoses against the backdrop of early germ theory debates. Importantly, these debates were themselves waged against a backdrop of social issues, including women's authority over their own bodies, the potential oversights of androcentric science, and the limits of certainty in a world saturated by empricism. Set in this carefully detailed context, the novel's ending tableau of solitude in fact represents a continued insistence on the need for a social world, in spite of its risks.

Each chapter of this book focuses on a different social issue as refracted through a different interpersonal relationship. As a precursor, the previous chapter focused on the broad social pressures that contagious outbreaks exert on large community bodies, along with authorial framing of these communities under pressure, which drew upon contemporary inoculation and vaccination debates. As I now turn to late-nineteenth-century texts, I will address more intimate, one-on-one relationships, which became capable of packaging more nuanced arguments about the ethics of community as germ theory and bacteriology became themselves more nuanced over time. The father-daughter relationship portrayed in *Washington Square* demonstrates quite nicely the instincts toward risk aversion that began to proliferate in this new era, counterbalanced against an omniscient narrative voice whose attitudes strikingly change across the course of the novel to highlight the hollowness of a life hermetically sealed against outside agents of risk and change. James uses this father-daughter unit as a microcosmic means of examining the gender relations at stake in the early germ theory debates, which centered on infected women's bodies and the potentially infectious obstetricians serving them.

By incorporating the burgeoning field of American obstetrics into his novel—the development of which was intimately intertwined with the eventual predominance of germ theory—James creates a case study through which to explore the minute effects scientific milieus have on the people who live within them. Indeed, alongside Lister's studies in general surgery and Pasteur's lab experiments, the field of obstetrics was, for a variety of reasons, at the epicenter of early germ theory debates. Beginning in the 1840s, statistical analysis of maternal mortality rates was specifically invoked by a handful of scientists to explain "childbed fever" (a postpartum disease also called puerperal fever, which was long recognized but increasing in prevalence at the time) as a contagious illness and therefore proof of the existence of organic germs that reproduce under certain conditions. Because the field of obstetrics met at the crossroads of several different women's issues—the marginalization of female-centered birthing experiences via midwives and the theorized increase in contagious deaths in parturient patients under obstetrical care, among others—this particular medical case study has much to say about human relationships and their tensile strength under biomedical pressures.

As an expatriate American, Henry James straddled the cultural tides affecting both sides of the Atlantic, making his work a unique viewpoint from which to consider transatlantic scientific developments. Such a perspective is critical to this study, since germ theory developed as a classic Kuhnian paradigm shift based on the slow accretions of the work of many practitioners and theorists around the world. *Washington Square* is one of James's few novels that takes place largely on American soil (making its transcontinental relevance quite apparent), and of all the texts covered in this study, it is the only one set at the beginning of the germ theory debates, in spite of its much later composition and publication dates contemporary with the period when bacteriology had already swung into high gear.[4] Given James's selection of a very specific time and place in germ theory's history, the novel's claims about bacteriological science and the human condition warrant careful attention. By reading the novel alongside developing germ theory debates, I resituate *Washington Square* within the historical and fiscal niche that James quite pointedly set it in and examine (as James did) this cultural milieu from the much-later scientific and social context of the novel's 1880 publication. Catherine's story is an important reminder that embodied and interpersonal experiences, made so apparent by disease, are also greatly dependent upon scientific understandings of disease and the body, which vary across time and are shaped by social biases to which all are subject.

Ian Bell has highlighted *Washington Square*'s temporal situation in the latter portion of the 1830s and early portion of the 1840s as a significant period in the history of American economic expansion.[5] Because James composed the novel at a chronological remove of nearly half a century, he was capable of examining the industrial and capitalistic growth during the 1830s and '40s in the light of his own age.[6] The period specified in *Washington Square*, "only slightly behind . . . the Gilded Age" in terms of American commercial growth, "signaled the development of a *national* economy and the consequential shift from self-sufficient farming and craft production to industrial manufacture and the factory system."[7] Indeed, *Washington Square* is set against a backdrop in which the narrator notes that "the murmur of trade had become a mighty uproar, which was music in the ears of all good citizens interested in . . . commercial development."[8]

Amid the commercial hum of the early decades of the nineteenth century, obstetrics arose as the first American medical specialty, and the field served as a lucrative market for doctors who could edge their way into this niche while simultaneously elbowing midwives out of it. Births were of course a nearly universal consequence of marriage in a time without reliable birth control, and the new specialists, obstetricians, were guaranteed a steady revenue stream in their practices. During the early parts of this century, doctors such as Austin Sloper realized that there was great potential for capital returns through investment in the sphere of childbirth, sparking a transition that gradually cast age-old terms such as *labor* and *delivery* with the neon-tinted lights of commerce. Later in the century—in the 1850s and '60s (just in between the time of the novel's setting and its composition)—a handful of doctors harnessed the force of the germ theory debates and brought it to bear upon this medico-fiscal metamorphosis, arguing that physicians' role in the birthing room contributed to increasing postpartum infection and death in this period.

James repurposes these gender-specific germ theory debates to retroactively assess the earlier forays of masculine practitioners into the once-feminine space of the birthing room. In doing so, James sets *Washington Square* up as a compelling case history vividly chronicling the social history of bias in science, made, as it is, by fallible humans subject to error and myopia. He then uses this retrospective assessment to warn readers away from normalizing the potentially negative implications of new scientific developments—in this case, the natural aversion to risk and risky encounters even after disastrous epidemics. In spite of these rather bleak themes, when read from between the interstices of this fiscal and scientific history, the novel incorporates a surprisingly optimistic conclusion that sketches out the potential for redemption and growth, even from within these systemic bounds.

The introductory paragraphs of *Washington Square* are an integral lens through which, I argue (as Bell also does), James intends the reader to view the rest of the novel. In the first three chapters—and largely in the first four paragraphs—James provides readers with important, systematically outlined details about the Slopers' occupations, life chronologies, and even the neighborhood where they live during the novel. As Bell notes, these preemptive descriptions—which pointedly *tell* rather than *show* important contingency data—are rather un-Jamesian. In fact, *Washington Square* "is the only novel for which James chose a specific locale as a title; [and] historical time and geographical place are the issues which overtly confront the reader to an extent insisted upon as nowhere else in James's works."[9]

The very first sentences of the novel, for instance, detail quite specifically the novel's timespan:

> During a portion of the first half of the present century, and more particularly during the latter part of it, there flourished and practiced in the city of New York a physician who enjoyed perhaps an exceptional share of the consideration which, in the United States, has always been bestowed upon the distinguished members of the medical profession.[10]

In only the second paragraph of the novel, the narrator in fact explains that Austin Sloper "had become a local celebrity" through his medical entrepreneurship, which "he cultivated . . . with . . . a definite . . . purpose."[11] In the United States, where, the narrator quickly notes, in order "to play a social part, you must either earn your income or make believe that you earn it," Austin Sloper has apparently made his name and fortune as "what is called a ladies' doctor."[12] Although the term "ladies' doctor" was sometimes used in periodicals to describe a wealthy doctor serving wealthy (often valetudinarian) women, this particular phrase was a relatively uncommon neologism, with no firmly solidified connotation. Given the specific temporal setting of *Washington Square* in the 1830s through the 1850s—a time of great growth in the obstetrical field—this malleable phrase easily slides into a gesture at the field of obstetrics, particularly since, by this time, wealthy American women increasingly chose to have their births presided over by obstetricians. At the very least, then, as a doctor to wealthy ladies, Austin Sloper's clients would have expected him to recommend a trusted colleague who specialized in obstetrics to attend them during childbirth.

Of Speculation and Speculums

It is generally agreed that by the mid-nineteenth century, obstetrician-assisted birth was an icon of fashion; most middle- and upper-class women were electing to have childbirth presided over by male doctors rather than female midwives.[13] For his part, Dr. Austin Sloper became a "local celebrity . . . who passed in the best society of New York,"[14] and so would have been physician to exactly the class of woman giving birth with obstetricians instead of midwives. Although, after some time, most of Dr. Sloper's patients come to be "overworked men of business," Austin's original interest in women's medical concerns make it clear early on that if he was not an obstetrician himself, he was certainly referring his clientele to a friend or colleague who was, and his patients, like any patient today, trusted his judgment and referral.[15]

All this James's narrator rushes to explain in only the first two paragraphs of the novel. However, in just the fourth paragraph, the narrator adds that Dr. Austin's first child, a son born prior to the opening of the story, died at three years of age "in spite of everything . . . *the father's science* could invent to save him."[16] Before the conclusion of the novel's first chapter, readers are presented with a man who represents the ostensibly omniscient glow of science sharply contrasted with the shadow of its failure in his own family. Two years afterward (still prior to the events that make up the novel), his wife bore another child, described simply as "an infant" whose "sex . . . rendered the poor child . . . an inadequate substitute for [the] lamented firstborn."[17] One week after this, Catherine's birth, her mother "suddenly betrayed alarming symptoms, and before another week had elapsed Austin Sloper was a widower."[18] The narrator reflects on Austin's losses:

> For a man whose trade was to keep people alive he had certainly done poorly in his own family. . . . Our friend, however, escaped criticism; that is, he escaped all criticism but his own. . . . He walked under the weight of this very private censure for the rest of his days.[19]

Although Austin personally takes some responsibility for his wife's and son's deaths, the cultural capital imbued by the "light" of science remains at the foreground of these early paragraphs. The narrator goes on to explain that Austin's reputation is so firmly established by this point that his practice is invulnerable to the potentially negative effects of these deaths. "Doctor Sloper had lost other patients besides the[se] two," the narrator qualifies, "which constituted an honorable precedent" according to "the world."[20] The deaths of his wife and son—and his involvement in their medical and obstetrical care is clearly indicated in this narrative sound bite of "the popular voice"—seem to the public to highlight a distanced, businesslike egalitarianism in practical methodology rather than a lapse of professional skill on his part.[21]

Dr. Sloper was not alone in working deliberately and assiduously to carve out commercial space for himself as a physician; all physicians in the nineteenth century had to act in much the same manner in order to achieve financial stability—a dynamic most clearly seen in those who aspired to improve their lot by hollowing out the obstetrical marketplace for themselves. Because midwives initially had some cultural sway, doctors in the early nineteenth century "had to eliminate midwives in order to protect their gateway to the whole practice."[22] However, "the doctors' answer to midwives' defenders was expressed not in terms of pecuniary motives but in terms of safety and the proper place of women."[23] The burgeoning authority of scientific knowledge in this period—which would reach its acme in the latter portions of the century from which James composed *Washington Square*—of course added heft to physicians' claims. Ultimately, doctors' efforts to corner the birthing market created a parturition culture where "maleness became a necessary attribute of safety, and femaleness became a condition in need of male medical control."[24]

By the time James composed *Washington Square*, obstetrics had firmly established its hold on the birthing market. From this late-century vantage point, a time steeped in bacteriology and well versed in germ theory, James could reflect on the changing dynamics of science and scientific knowledge in the nineteenth century—specifically as it was refracted against the crosscutting factor of gender. Equipped with the tools of the trade (forceps, anesthetics, speculums, prying fingers, and a diploma), doctors had systematically pushed midwives to the margins of medical necessity and prestige.[25] As one obstetrician, Walter Channing, famously noted, the physician "must do something. He cannot remain a spectator merely, where there are many witnesses."[26] Indeed, the very presence of invented tools and instruments allowed doctors to create for themselves an identity as men who "did something" (to restate Channing's words, reproduced as the epigraph to this chapter). This ability to "do things" with tools and claims to scientific truth allowed doctors to proclaim their utility over midwives.[27] This trend was kept in continued momentum by the development of later obstetrical techniques, drugs, and invasive use of the obstetrician's hands. Dr. Sloper is specifically described as a practitioner who subscribed to this *modus operandi*; although he is a "scholarly doctor," the narrator is quick to prevent the reader from assuming that there is anything "abstract in [Sloper's] remedies—he always ordered you to take something."[28] Additionally, although his wife came to him with quite a fortune, the narrator confidently asserts that this "made no difference in the [professional] line he had traced for himself," stating moreover that his "purpose had not been *preponderantly* to make money—it had been rather to learn something and to *do* something."[29] True to Channing's and James's turn of phrase, Wertz and Wertz explain that

[e]ven though well-educated physicians recognized that . . . instruments could be dangerous, in their practice they also had to appear to *do* something. . . . The doctor could not appear to be indifferent or inattentive or useless. He had to establish his identity by doing something.[30]

Ignasz Semmelweis and Statistical Assessment of Maternal Mortality Rates

Ironically, it was this very insistence on "doing" that resulted in skyrocketing maternal mortality rates in precisely this same period.[31] Because of the rise of empiricism in hospital medicine at the time, obstetricians, unlike midwives, often traveled from autopsy cadavers to the birthing room. Ignasz Semmelweis put his empiricist training to task on this broader hospital practice, and theorized that it was responsible for rising maternal mortality. In the 1840s, he began to meticulously record epidemiological data trends from maternity wards, concluding that obstetricians themselves were carrying infection to parturient mothers from autopsies performed on other women who had died of postpartum infection. Semmelweis's research showed that hospital wards run by midwives had lower rates of puerperal fever than those run by doctors, even when the former were more overcrowded, and illustrated furthermore that when doctors cleaned their hands with a chlorinated lime solution between patients, maternal mortality dropped from around 10 percent to rates comparable with midwives'—closer to 3.5 percent.[32] For reasons that are unclear, Semmelweis did not publish his findings in writing until nearly1860. He did ultimately lose positions because of disagreement with his findings, so it is quite possible that he was aware of the controversy it would ignite. Nevertheless, the medical community that surrounded him in Vienna was at the forefront of the medical field as a whole and did much to promote his work. A handful of his colleagues even went so far as to publish parts of his findings for him, and they did much to promote the circulation of his ideas by electing him as a representative speaker in public debates—the existence of which are testament to the publicity which the subject received—on the topic of the contagiousness of puerperal fever.

Cultivating and growing the field of obstetrics meant that doctors had to proclaim their own value over midwives. Therefore, perceived credibility was of the utmost importance for doctors who wanted to edge their way into the birthing market. For these reasons, among others, many in the medical profession violently argued against Semmelweis's findings.[33] In some respects, it is pure happenstance that the early germ theory debates began in the highly gendered arena of the birthing room presided over by male doctors. One major factor was simply the availability and apparent presence of visible data. The women dying of puerperal fever were in a stable location rather than out in the community, and so statistics were readily calculated based on a known sample size. Additionally, puerperal fever was both highly recognizable and highly contagious. Epidemiological trends are more apparent to the casual observer when a disease is highly virulent. That is, a disease that easily transfers from one person to another is simply more obviously infectious at the macroscopic level. The previous chapter on plague demonstrates this; the subsequent chapter on tuberculosis (which is quite difficult to contract) demonstrates the opposite. Group A streptococcal infections such as puerperal fever (most well known in its phenotypic manifestation as strep throat today) are easily contracted and have quick incubation periods, and thus its contagious nature was simply quite visible to some doctors working in maternity wards. As Defoe's and Shelley's texts helpfully demonstrate, the notion that some diseases were contagious was not new. However, its growth as a predominant mode by which disease was conceptualized *was* new to the Victorian era, and it began precisely in this period, when obstetricians moved into the birthing field and a handful of them began to notice what they believed to be contagious infections sweeping through labor and delivery wards.

The presence of a particular doctor such as Semmelweis, poised with a particular type of empirical training and given a post in a particular ward destined to be full of infection, may have been coincidental (Semmelweis had in fact applied to a number of other medical specializations before this; obstetrics was his last resort). However, the very public, often very vitriolic debates surrounding the contagiousness of puerperal fever took hold and gained momentum precisely because they occurred in this gendered space, where patriarchal authority had much at stake in the outcome of the debate. These debates about a specific infection came to represent the wider question of germ theory altogether. Moreover, as both sides of this debate were comprised of male medical professionals, both arguing for the credibility of their profession (either the anticontagionists' previous and continued infallibility, or the new and current infallibility of the contagionists), germ theory gained publicity in the popular press by proxy as it served as the vehicle for larger debates regarding male authority over female bodies.

As with Virchow and Koch's disagreement over germ theory mentioned in the introduction (Virchow's reluctance having less to do with empirical disagreement than with his concern over the fallout of highlighting *people* as carriers of disease), and as Science and Technology Studies (STS) has helpfully elucidated in recent years, it is reductive to think about medical and scientific debates in terms of the ignorant and the correct parties. Indeed, the present book would be doing but little service to the field of STS to which it owes so much if it accepted germ theory at face value as somehow more enlightened than earlier theories. As indicated by my introduction, I intend to do no such thing, and if anything, the opposite. It is tempting at times, however, to view Semmelweis's and Holmes's opponents as maliciously unwilling to acknowledge their complicity in rampant female mortality. It is tempting, in fact, because these are the rhetorical terms in which Semmelweis and Holmes (and others among them) couched their side of the debate. Semmelweis's 1859 *The Etiology, Concept, and Prophylaxis of Childbed Fever,* for instance, is reported matter-of-factly and shows great attention to detail. However, even his carefully annotated quantitative data analysis breaks down at times into bleak despair as he calls for physicians to acknowledge their involvement in maternal death:

> I must affirm that only God knows the number of patients who went prematurely to their graves because of me. . . . No matter how painful and oppressive such a recognition [of doctors' role in women's deaths] may be, the remedy does not lie in suppression. If the misfortune is not to persist forever, then the truth must be made known to everyone concerned.

Oliver Wendell Holmes: Pathos, Applied to Statistics

In America, Oliver Wendell Holmes worked for the same goals as Semmelweis, insisting upon the contagious nature of puerperal fever and urging doctors to adopt aseptic and antiseptic methods, though his arguments were structured on theoretical reasoning rather than empirical methods, and therefore caused less of a stir.[34] He was a vocal supporter of Semmelweis and promoted his works in the American context, but tended more toward impassioned rhetorical pleas than scrutiny of data. While Semmelweis's studies were groundbreaking, and his name is still taught in medical schools today, Holmes had perhaps a keener awareness of what science journalists know today: the lay public is quickly bored of tables and graphs. Holmes tapped into the human element of the equation, supporting it when necessary with Semmelweis's data, and in doing so, brought the urgency of the debates to the American shores. His famous essay, "The Contagiousness of Puerperal Fever," thusly opens by situating himself as a mediator between the lay public and the scientific profession, a meta-analyst capable of translating and explaining findings and their significance to the public. He begins by acknowledging the intensity of disagreement that characterized the puerperal fever debates, but adding, in a tone rhetorically aimed to showcase his skill at deescalating hot-button issues, that "whatever apprehensions and beliefs were entertained [by the public] . . . a fuller knowledge of the facts would be acceptable to all present."[35] He continues by adding that he has striven to find "the best records . . . [and] . . . the most trustworthy practitioners . . . to learn what experience had to teach in the matter, and arrived at the results contained" in his study.[36] Throughout his paper, his claims indeed *rest* on data-driven evidence, but *appeal* through pathos. "The subject of this Paper," he says, "has the same profound interest for me at the present moment as it had when I was first collecting the terrible evidence," and he continues on to emotionally note his uncertainty as to whether "I shall ever again have so good an opportunity of being useful as was granted me by the raising of the question which produced this Essay."[37] Holmes built upon Semmelweis, then, in important ways directed at appealing to broad listeners and readers in the American public, and he was thusly a rhetorically minded extension of Semmelweis in America, responsible for a great deal of publicity regarding the findings in that context.

Mansplaining: Victorian Edition

The opponents of both men were equally as impassioned; at their harshest, many were openly hostile to claims about the contagiousness of puerperal fever by publicly refusing to wash their hands after autopsy and before delivery simply to argue their point. Even at their gentlest, these arguments took on a patronizing tone typical of nineteenth-century Angel of the House discourse. However, given Semmelweis's ten-year delay in publishing his findings, it is possible to read him as operating from the same sort of problematic male savior complex as his opponents, with merely different unquestioned motivations. Indeed, as often as their opponents spoke in patronizing tones about women's bodies and their own exalted role as physician-protector, doctors such as Semmelweis and Holmes cast themselves as women's vigilante heroes, arriving just in time to rescue the collective damsels in distress from mustache-twirling anticontagionists. One could ask, for instance, that if he felt so strongly about saving women's lives, why did he wait an entire decade to publish his findings and lend credibility to his claims? Such issues of motive are impossible to fully know, and it is therefore more helpful to simply assert that regardless of reductive terms such as *right* and *wrong,* and irrespective of who, if anyone, was more sincerely selfless in championing women's issues, the battleground became such a vocal battleground, so highly publicized in the public eye, *because it was about* women—and, regardless of camps and sides, almost always involved men making claims about women's bodies and health. Thus, women's issues and issues of gender and sexuality were early on deeply intertwined in subjective and actively evolving understandings of germ theory, disease, and the body.

The gendered nature of this debate itself resulted in its intense tenor in print, an intensity that I would argue lent interest and popular circulation to the claims of germ theory in its infancy. A topic that might otherwise have been relegated to the back pages of scientific miscellany instead became one of the key issues of the day.

Even the more tempered of the anticontagionist responses to the puerperal fever germ theory debates smacked, as I have said, of a patronizing tone that was easy to read as a disregard for the urgency of the matter. Hugh L. Hodge, for instance, argues:

> It has been suggested that, as the question is yet undetermined, the patient should have the benefit of the doubt, and be informed of the danger; but we have just seen that this would not be for her benefit. The moment she doubts, or even speculates, she is in danger; her fears are excited, and in spite even of reason and common sense, her mind will be disturbed, her susceptibilities will be augmented, and her powers of endurance diminished. It is far more humane, as well as reasonable, to keep her in happy ignorance of danger.[38]

This was a common argument—that women needed to be protected by doctors from their own potentially deadly fears, which were more dangerous than puerperal fever itself. Holmes and Semmelweis responded with verve, pathos, and at times outright aggression against these men. The periodical evidence of their debates comes as close to tabloid-level sensationalism as is perhaps possible for scientific treatises.

After quoting Hodge in his epigraph as an example of problematic anti-contagionist discourse, Holmes, in his famous essay "On the Contagiousness of Childbed Fever," proceeds to say that he would rather continue to reiterate his point "though it should call out a hundred [such] counterblasts, proving to the satisfaction of their authors that [he had] proved nothing" (Holmes, 106). He continues: "[F]or my part, I had rather rescue one mother from being poisoned by her attendant, than claim to have saved forty out of fifty patients to whom I carried the disease" (ibid.). This statement exemplifies the male savior complex embedded in both sides of this argument: Holmes states that he would rather save only one life while proving himself right than to save forty women in the act of being theoretically incorrect in his masculine sphere of medical science. His use of the word *rescue* similarly invokes the chivalric white knight as a structuring device for this claim. Importantly, Holmes's weighing of one life against forty also prefigures Austin Sloper's actuarial-style risk assessments and utter risk aversion, which are the ultimate biopolitical ramifications of germ theory's isolationist ideology.

Semmelweis personally undertook a letter-writing campaign directed at anyone who was unconvinced by his findings. Again, while it was indeed often probably true to note that doctors were reluctant to accept Semmelweis's findings because they highlighted male oversight and ignorance, Semmelweis's response (like Holmes's) is not to argue for data alone, but to rhetorically cast himself as women's savior and solution to the problem at large. "This murder must cease," he begins in one letter, "and in order that the murder ceases *I* will keep watch," figuring himself as the singular white knight of women's justice in a world of darkness.[39] In another letter, he increases his charge: "[Y]our doctrine . . . is based on the corpses of puerperal women murdered out of ignorance."[40] He continues: "[S]hould you . . . continue to train your pupils [incorrectly], I declare before God and the world that you are a murderer."[41] In another letter, he disparages contemporary medical licensing, saying that even in new, cutting-edge facilities "a great deal can be accomplished with regard to murder, if one only possesses the necessary qualifications."[42] His repeated use of the term *murderer* modernizes the chivalric imagery of his letters, casting himself now as an agent of justice.

Alongside Pasteur's highly publicized experiments in France and Lister's in England, the debates over postpartum infection were undoubtedly some of the most important events that gave space in the popular imagination and mindset for germ theory to take precedence—and the emotional tone of everyone involved in these debates lent excitement, interest, and therefore wide social engagement to the new disease cosmology. Their prominent role in periodical publications brought about vast changes in medical procedure on the whole, which, while serving to effectively curb maternal mortality rates, were not without the biopolitical consequences that are at issue in this book. That is, in finding ways to control and reduce deaths from contaminants, Victorians then sallied forth with hyperbolic zeal for antisepsis and quarantine away from risk encounters (recall Holmes's one over forty fantasy) that form the basis for the countercultural movement I note in each chapter of this book, and that are specifically outlined in *Washington Square*.

Only because of the quickly circulated and widely read nature of these debates between the 1840s and '60s could an 1890s midwifery book open with such gusto:

> The practice of obstetric medicine has, during the last few years, undergone a stupendous change. The two great revolutionary and epoch-making forces of modern medicine, anesthetics and antiseptics, have in no branch of the healing art exercised a greater influence than in obstetrics and gynaecology. But lately, the subject of child-bed fever was enveloped in Egyptian darkness. Nothing can more pointedly show the hopelessness of the situation less than forty years ago, than the following quotation from the writings of a distinguished American obstetrician of that period. He says, "I prefer to attribute them" (that is, cases of puerperal fever) "to accident or Providence, of which I can form a conception, rather than to a contagion of which I cannot form any clear idea, at least, as to this particular malady."[43]

When James's narrator tells readers in 1880, then, in just the fourth paragraph of *Washington Square* that Dr. Austin Sloper's wife died in the 1840s after childbirth and within the specific incubation period unique to childbed fever, he has instantly shuttled his audience into the thick of debates entangled with hot-button issues such as medical professionalization, scientific paradigm shifts, and the potential for women's mistreatment at the hands of men. The scientific context of the novel reveals what its anticlimactic plot belies as mere character study. The stakes in *Washington Square* are high, they are intense, and they would have been vividly apparent to any nineteenth-century reader who had lived through the period in which the novel was set.

Risk Encounters and Their Discontents

Like so many women just before and during the early germ theory debates, Dr. Sloper's wife died of puerperal fever. As I've mentioned, in the opening pages of *Washington Square* James is immediately and meticulously specific about a few things: the time period in which the story takes place, the wealthy economic status of the Slopers, and the precise incubation and symptomatic period of Mrs. Sloper just before her death. For an author made famous by long books of character study that "tell the truth at a slant," as it were, these concrete details stand out, more so because they appear in the opening paragraphs of a novel in place of more typical, musing character or landscape description. Thus, James focuses his reader's attention early on to the fact that Mrs. Sloper was a wealthy woman who would have had a medicalized birth in the period of the 1840s, precisely when medicalized births tended to kill women with infection in the postpartum period. Indeed, puerperal fever was quite recognizable and obvious to most practitioners, even if its etiology was a matter of contention. To cite just one example, an old French proverb indicates the precise two-to-nine-day incubation period of the infection: "heaven stays open nine days for the woman in childbed."[44] This is precisely how Mrs. Sloper presents, when, "a week after [Catherine's] birth," she "suddenly betray[s] alarming symptoms" and dies shortly thereafter.[45]

The narrator insists that Austin Sloper's business did not decline as a result of his wife's and son's deaths. Yet Austin's apparent guilt after his wife's death, coupled with the family's temporal and economic context outlined early in the novel, suggests his subsequent awareness that he had thrown his lot in with the losing side of the germ theory debates in his choice of an obstetrician for his wife. In a general sense, given the widespread myopia (voluntary or otherwise) of physicians as to their role in rampant maternal death, enterprising obstetricians and physicians like Austin who promoted their use in effect functioned much like stock or land speculators, hazarding their best guesses as to what sorts of investments of time, energy, and, in this case, medical protocol would yield the best results in terms of profits and client outcomes. Indeed, during the period in which *Washington Square* is set, stock and land speculation was on the rise, and both, like obstetrics, were considered "an acceptable means to wealth . . . emphasiz[ing] further the anonymity of developing capitalism."[46] When Austin loses his wife, then, he has effectively lost out in a bad investment and is thusly situated in this text as the tropological figure (so common in Victorian fiction) of a wealthy man who has lost everything due to bad speculation. However, the narrative voice is quick to divest readers of the supposition that Austin's loss in speculation was financial. Austin's guilt, then, coupled with the fact that readers learn simultaneously that his business did not suffer, means that Austin's "loss" in speculation was emotional and personal rather than financial. His wager in the then-uncertain science around germ theory and parturient bodies in the obstetrical field led directly to his speculation that his wife was safe, either in his or in one of his colleagues' professional hands during childbirth, a gamble which leaves him with a permanent deficit.[47]

From these first paragraphs of the novel, then, the narrative voice primes readers to conflate—for the sake of James's allegory—fiscal and filial risk. Doctor Sloper represents the economic speculation hazarded by obstetricians, and his parallel trajectory as a successful medical businessman is negatively correlated with the dwindling size of his family after the loss of his son and his wife. This story's very opening represents a crucible, whereupon Austin does an ideological about-face. His loss through speculative allegiance with the anticontagionists leads to his problematic flight from community risk encounters. He now espouses the logical conclusions of germ theory: aseptic isolation and a life hermetically sealed from risk. He imposes this upon his only remaining filial connection, Catherine, when she wants to marry Morris. Austin is well aware that Morris is a likely fortune hunter, and what in many ways seems to be his overbearing protectiveness throughout the novel can simultaneously be read as his compulsive maintenance of Catherine in a hermetically sealed environment, never to be speculated—that is, cast out into the environment of uncertain results. Again, this risk hazarding is equal parts financial—for her marriage would expose her impressive fortune to misuse and depletion by her husband—and personal, as any marriage comes with uncertain emotional fates. Austin's seemingly natural paternal protection, then, walks in lockstep with his traumatic response to risk and failed speculation in his earlier life.

Significantly, it is only after the events described in the novel's opening pages, outlining the speculations that left Austin without two-thirds of his original filial assets, that readers are privy to Austin's interactions with Catherine. Moreover, by the time the novel opens, Austin has not just lost two-thirds of his investment: he has lost the *more important* two-thirds, the male child and the individual capable of producing more children. Read in this light, Dr. Sloper's ostensibly concerned protection of Catherine from her (likely) mercenary suitor Morris Townsend—who is, interestingly, a speculator in women through marriage and a land speculator by trade—take on a different hue. His jealous guarding of her is, rather, revealed as a zealous ideological shift toward risk aversion. He does not simply refuse to accept her desire to marry Morris. He imposes upon Catherine a life of antiseptic protection from risk through the only possible means—total isolation from a social world in which every choice and interaction is necessarily speculated upon a sea of chances, bodies, and events.

His ambivalent treatment of her, however, results from the fact that she is a living reminder of his failed speculation and the risks of, well, risk. Instead of having a wife, a son, and a daughter, he has Catherine—a metonymic reminder of both the absence of the former two and of the catastrophic consequences a single decision can have upon our innately uncertain, tortuous, mystifying lives. The first description of Catherine in the entire novel comes from Austin's point of view, and again underscores a relationship winnowed down to a cost-benefit analysis: "[H]is little girl remained to him; and though she was not what he had desired, he proposed to make himself make the best of her."[48] Dr. Sloper bitterly regards Catherine as an unsatisfactory return on his failed endeavor. He can never shake the feeling, given this, that Catherine "ha[s] played him a trick."[49] Waiting for the perfect moment of risk-free speculation, Austin forces Catherine to live a stagnant life with him, as he waits to assess the perfect suitor for her, one who brings to the table no risk whatsoever.

As we have seen from the previous chapter, the authors I cover here tend to take a paradoxically radical stance on this issue, insisting on what is of course an undeniable truth of existence. That is, using disease as a vehicle to further their claims that nothing is risk-free and no outcomes can be perfectly controlled or predicted, they connect this notion to its logical, but generally repressed, conclusion: to attempt to avoid risk is therefore a hollow victory of isolation and paranoia while it lasts, and is ultimately useless. Austin's aversion to seemingly bad investments (in terms of husbands) and his search for a risk-free connection for Catherine are akin to the Black Spectre and the dying grandmother in Shelley's *The Last Man.* All of these characters serve only to demonstrate the futility of self-protective isolation from risk. As I mentioned in the introduction, even the new science of germ theory did nothing if not demonstrate to Victorians that germs were everywhere, pervading all of the atmosphere, inhaled and exhaled with every breath, and physically connecting everyone in a sea of microbial trails. Our very human attempts at avoiding connection to others on this microscopic level—as demonstrated literarily through macroscopic human endeavors at isolation—can never fully succeed. These notions are based on the illusory idea that there is any way to avoid the fact that we *are* connected to our fellow man, even if only through the atmosphere we breathe, and generally through much more. Isolation and quarantine, as Defoe so early on urged, only result in delaying the inevitable at best, or an explosive overflow and frenzied human attempts to escape even self-imposed quarantine at worst. As we shall see, Austin's interactions with Catherine result in this overflow, as she rebels against his stifling efforts to hermetically seal her off from risky encounters. Paradoxically, this is because, since Austin figures her in his own mind as nothing more than the metonymic reminder of his failed speculations, she therefore never comes to embody anything more human and relational for him. Instead, she remains for him a dehumanized figure of the catastrophic potential of risky endeavors. As Austin rejects Morris as a suitor and searches out more suitable ones, Catherine embodies through-out the novel both precisely what she represents to him through his past investment and all she can represent to him in the present—an asset waiting to be liquidated, with her own potential for output of goods by way of children, if the right investor (by way of a husband) comes along.

In spite of Austin's cold, pecuniary attitudes toward Catherine, it is hard to deny that he was probably correct in his assessment of her suitor: Morris *was* most likely marrying Catherine for her money. However, this was not truly at issue for Dr. Sloper. Much more important than Morris's intentions were his risk factors—Morris was an unwise speculation. Austin states as much in no uncertain terms to Morris himself:

> [Y]our absence of means, of a profession, of visible resources or prospects, places you in a category from which it would be imprudent for me to select a husband for my daughter, who is a weak young woman with a large fortune. In any other capacity I am perfectly prepared to like you. As a son-in-law, I abominate you.[50]

It is absolutely Morris's lack of money and not his daughter's future happiness that is on Austin's mind, for he further qualifies his statement to Morris by adding that "even if [Catherine] were not weak, you would still be a penniless man."[51] Austin specifically implicates Catherine's mental weakness here, as the narrator is at great pains in the early portions of the novel to point out Catherine's "robust, healthy and well-grown" constitution.[52] Since she is adamantly described as quite capable of good, effective childbearing, James further highlights Austin's interest in shuttling her off to the proper man. It is not her physical weakness that is problematic for the production of proper heirs and a return on Austin's investment; quite the opposite—it is her perceived mental *inability* to select a proper man with whom to mate and *provide* this return on Austin's investment. Austin deems Catherine incapable of making her own risk assessments, and so he attempts to control agents of risk and their access to her, keeping her effectively quarantined in his home and under his guard. Again, the scientific and fiscal intertwine in a feverish torrent of calculated risk as Austin's reads his potential profit gains in light of his assumption that Catherine will be unsuccessful at independent Darwinian natural selection. Austin repeatedly insists, for instance, on taxonomically describing Morris's situation as an undesirable "category."[53]

Though he admits that Morris's situation is "but an accident," he asserts that his "thirty years' medical practice" has shown him "that accidents may have far-reaching consequences."[54] The accidental death of his wife and child at the hands of his masculine, scientific authority stripped him of all he had invested in the market of filial connection—aside from Catherine, that is. With her as his only potential investment, he refuses to lose what little equity he believes she has by making another risky speculation—that of accepting an impoverished husband as an investor in his daughter. James deftly illustrates Austin's focus on the potential financial investment of Catherine by depicting subsequent marriage proposals that he approves of from both "a widower, a man with a genial temperament, *a handsome fortune,* and three little girls" and "a young lawyer, who, *with the prospect of a great practice,* and the reputation of a most agreeable man, had had the shrewdness . . . to believe that she would suit him better than several younger and prettier girls."[55] Austin is a man of business, and he quickly encourages the efforts of both of these men, regardless of Catherine's feelings toward them. He "advise[s] [the lawyer] to persevere" in his pursuit of Catherine, for instance, in spite of her lack of interest in the man.[56] Catherine's feelings certainly do not motivate Austin's choices for her. Austin has waited carefully for a chance to invest what is his capital by default only, and Morris is hardly the chance he has been looking for.

Intriguingly, Catherine's own actions in the novel are a rejection of the patriarchal thinking, and more importantly, the risk-averse calculations that her father embodies. Catherine has only a few options in response to her father's demands that she detach herself from Morris. She can elope, thus directly defying his wishes, or she can obey her father and give up her emotional attachment for Morris, thereby securing her financial inheritance. She might even marry a subsequent suitor, as her father wishes, to make up for her loss. All of these options, however, exemplify extremist and impossibly unrealistic responses to risk encounters. I've already demonstrated authorial responses to the idea that avoiding risk entirely is at all possible. As will become clear directly, the narrator of *Washington Square* ultimately aligns the novel's moral compass with Catherine by its conclusion, so her refusal to remain hermetically sealed from risk is cast as positive in the text. Yet as I've said in my introduction, and as I will continue to insist, refusing to live a life of isolated, risk-free quarantine does not, of course, mean martyred pursuit of infection and death. That is, as much as refusal to marry Morris or marrying a subsequent "risk-free" suitor are unrealistic attempts at quarantine from risk, to marry him would be to knowingly encounter ruin. By about midway through the novel, Morris's motivations become clear, for he absconds into the night after she agrees to marry him without her fortune. When he returns years later, Catherine is far from willing to sacrifice herself on the altar of old affections, risk acceptance, *or,* importantly, to the mere principle of defying her father. As Austin himself muses, Catherine's reactions to Morris are

> extremely mixed up, and the mixture is extremely odd. It will produce some third element, and that's what I'm waiting to see. I wait with suspense—with positive excitement; and that is a sort of emotion that I didn't suppose Catherine would ever provide for me.[57]

As we will see, this "third element" will be, unbeknownst to him, Catherine's surprising disavowal of the two, more obvious binary options of obeying or eloping (read: asepsis or infectious death) that circle around the men in her life. Instead, she embraces a third, personally determined option both between and outside of these two poles. Through strategic invocation of the figure of the male obstetrician and early germ theory debates at the beginning of *Washington Square*, James reveals by its conclusion that all of the choices readily available to Catherine inevitably circumscribe her in a world of male dominion, and that a seemingly anticlimactic ending is her only way out of its stifling bounds. And the linchpin of the novel is Catherine's burgeoning awareness of this fact.

She awakens to the reality that all of the men in her world, through their attempt to mitigate risk for themselves, in fact make Catherine the object of their speculations. This is particularly ironic when it comes to Austin, who is so motivated by a desire never to speculate on outcomes again that he is apparently unaware that he does almost nothing *but* speculate on Catherine's actions and reactions. This self-fulfilling return of the repressed demonstrates further James's point that there are no fully predictable outcomes—everything involves some amount of risk and uncertainty.

As an inadvertent speculator on Catherine's choices, while Austin Sloper often expresses intense rage in response to Catherine's unrelenting affection for Morris, he equally as often expresses intense excitement at the idea that Catherine will disobey him and elope with Morris. His first assertion that he believes Catherine "will stick" (i.e., maintain her feelings for Morris) is spoken with a "comical" element, as it offers Austin some "prospect of entertainment."[58] In speaking with his sister about Catherine's situation later, he compares himself and his speculations about Catherine and Morris to an unrelenting "geometrical proposition."[59] In fact, he refers to Catherine and Morris as geometrical "surfaces" of which he has "taken . . . measure."[60] True to form, Austin's fantasies of this sort are always and unequivocally imaged in scientific and mathematical terms. Catherine's feelings are merely so many actuarial equations for Austin and nothing more, and he never allows for the possibility that his daughter might interest him through a surprising exhibition of her ability to act autonomously and outside of his speculations about her. In this, at least, he shares a quality with the man he sees as his rival. Morris, too, thinks of Catherine in calculated terms of chance and probability. Even in conversations with one another during which the men argue about their divergent plans for her future, they both agree on their conceptualization of her as a formula of probability to be manipulated and the result to be speculated upon. During one such conversation, for instance, Morris defiantly asks Austin: "Are you sure your daughter will give me up?"[61] Austin proudly replies that he has a "great fund of respect and affection . . . to draw upon," making him confident in her obedience.[62] "I, too, have a fund of affection to draw upon," Morris retorts—arguing his own point but accepting and maintaining Austin's assessment of Catherine's emotions as financial algorithms to be worked out mathematically and pragmatically.[63]

On his own, as well, Morris conceptualizes Catherine mathematically. The opening of chapter 22 is comprised of Morris's speculation of his potential outcomes with Catherine. To marry her would be to gain a wife but to lose her father's dowry; to give her up would be to lose the opportunity of gaining at least the inheritance she is due from her mother. He determines to hold out for the entire inheritance, because "with his fine parts he rated himself high, and he had a perfectly definite appreciation of his value, which seemed to him inadequately represented by the sum" of the mother's fortune alone.[64] As he continues to consider his chances of successfully obtaining *all* of Catherine's potential fortune, he acknowledges to himself that

> Doctor Sloper's opposition was the unknown quantity in the problem he had to work out. The natural way to work it out was by marrying Catherine; but in mathematics there are many shortcuts, and Morris was not without a hope that he should yet discover one.[65]

Like Austin, Morris never calculates Catherine's potential for independent thought and action as a variable in his equations.

All of this mental math—of which Catherine is the object—comes after a conversation Morris has with Catherine's aunt, who works to promote the match between the two throughout the plot. Morris dislikes the woman but tolerates her because he needs her assistance. While the two are talking during this particular scene, the aunt claims that Austin has threatened to throw her out of his home because of her meddling and implies that this would leave her destitute. Morris is skeptical of this statement—he "had a speculative idea that she had a little property; but he naturally did not press this."[66] Although for a moment the humming gears of mathematic calculation digress and tally up the value of a woman other than Catherine, the consistently iterated theme of the novel shows up here like a nightmarish coda: the men in the novel persistently calculate the value of women as actuarial risk factors, evaluating their various qualities mindlessly and nearly automatically, as if these calculations were natural. Critical representations of women as dowry-commodities were hardly novel in nineteenth-century fiction. However, James expands his marriage market critique by addressing marriage's frequent outcome in an age devoid of effective contraception: childbirth, potential postpartum infection, and the obstetrician who had come to speculate in this realm of risk and antiseptic obviation.

Both Austin and Morris box Catherine in with their "speculative ideas" about her and what she will do—and both see her independence as limited by a choice of obedience to one or the other of them. To obey her father or to marry Morris both dead-end in a male-dominated world. Defying her father and eloping with Morris would in fact confirm his belief that her subjective emotional experiences can be contained by a set of actuarial postulates and solution sets. Equally so, of course, it becomes increasingly clear that eloping with Morris would mean subjecting herself to embracing obvious ruin with open arms merely to defy her father's antiseptic, isolationist practices. Toward the conclusion of the novel, Catherine begins to distance herself from her father, and it is this separation that begins to allow her some autonomy. Austin mentions Morris one day while contemplating what he accurately believes to be his own impending death. When he asks her to promise never to marry Morris, Catherine simply responds by saying, "I don't think I can promise that."[67] Her father reasserts his request several times, mentioning that compliance is the perquisite for inclusion in his will. When Catherine firmly sticks to her original answer, he finally asks for an explanation. Catherine responds evasively, simply saying, "I can't explain . . . and I can't promise."[68] By refusing her father a concrete answer—something that smacks of the supposed objectivity found in actuarial tables and risk avoidance—she marks the final refusal of her participation in a world defined by risk calculation and safety through social isolation. A year later, upon finding that she has, indeed, been largely excluded from her father's will, Catherine claims to "like [the will] very much."[69] Through her resistance to both her father and Morris, Catherine has in fact secured, in her very exclusion from the will, the ability to live outside of a devitalizing life that values personal risk avoidance over life-giving encounters with others, risky though they may be.[70]

Catherine's Paradoxical Transcendence

Paradoxically, then, by choosing self-imposed isolation, Catherine sidesteps precisely the ideological aversion to risky encounters with other bodies that Morris and her father advocate. By resisting all the options placed before her by calculating men—by doing the one thing none of them predict—Catherine proves false their sense that interpersonal relationships in all their risky messiness are something that can be speculated upon and predicted. Surrounded by options that begin and end in male speculative authority (doctor, father, husband, suitor, lover), Catherine slowly embarks upon a plan of resistance throughout the novel. Beginning with her resistance to Morris's first appeals, she initially refuses to defy her father, thereby resisting Morris's speculation that her passion for his masculinity will overpower her better judgment. By making it clear to her father that she refuses to rid herself of affection for Morris, she resists both her father's control and his assumption that female emotions are mechanized forces to be trained, shaped, and controlled by a proper set of calculated formulae.

By the novel's end, Catherine breaks free from Austin's superimposed definitions of her as dull, plain, and uninteresting, and asserts herself as an emotional, capable, independent being *through* her resistance of all the options the male world has provided to her. She refuses to relinquish her autonomy to Morris by eloping with him. She refuses to allow her father to control or assume the very possibility of the mechanization of her inner, subjective experiences. As mentioned earlier, when Austin realizes he cannot control her feelings, he turns to packaging them into neat files of scientific postulates, subject to his experimentation and observation. At this stage, he becomes less concerned with what seems to be his actively failing personal agenda and more with his bare ability to assess her decision-making processes from a speculative, mathematical standpoint. Throughout the latter portions of the novel, she refuses to conform to his reactionary postulation of her emotional world and "averts herself rigidly from the *idea* of marrying other people," even while she no longer pursues Morris.[71]

As a nonparticipant, Catherine is free from any ties that fetter her to a world of male interaction, which, for her, inevitably stacks the deck against women by allowing not for *inter*action but only for subjugation, production, and mechanized action. Ergo, a seemingly anticlimactic ending in which Catherine quietly lives in her father's virtually empty house for the rest of her life suddenly becomes a regenerative, self-affirming one—an ending that reaffirms, counterintuitively, the value of community and the devitalizing nature of purity through hermetically sealed isolation via her rejection of others' definitions of what that community life should look like. By the end of her story, Catherine's awareness of the true nature of the men in her life catalyzes her growth and allows her to participate in society on her terms. Her awareness of their speculations about her is always discussed alongside her increasing agency in the story:

> From her own point of view the great facts of her career were that Morris Townsend had trifled with her affection, and that her father had broken its spring. Nothing could ever alter these facts; they were always there, like her name, her age, her plain face. Nothing could ever undo the wrong or cure the pain that Morris had inflicted on her, and nothing could ever make her feel toward her father as she felt in her younger years. There was something dead in her life, and her duty was to fill the void. Catherine recognized this duty to the utmost; she had a great disapproval of brooding and moping. . . . She mingled freely in

the usual gaieties of town, and she became at last an inevitable figure at all respectable entertainments. She was greatly liked, and as time went on, she grew to be a sort of kindly maiden aunt to the younger portion of society. Young girls were apt to confide to her their love affairs . . . and young men to be fond of her without knowing why.[72]

As a nonparticipant in risk-speculative culture, Catherine finds freedom and room for self-actualization in other parts of her community, which she identifies and enters into of her own volition. And it is the narrator who allows space for the astute reader to see Catherine not as the unfulfilled, sexually repressed spinster that predominant cultural norms might code her as, but rather as the vibrant, self-fulfilled woman she has become through resistance to participation in parts of culture that cast humans as actuarial entries.

The narrator provides this window because, presumably male, he aligns himself in every way with Austin Sloper's view of Catherine at the novel's opening. Indeed, Catherine, Austin, and the narrator all seem to agree on a few points at the beginning of the novel—Catherine is quiet, shy, mousy, dull, uninteresting, unintelligent, untalented, and with very little taste.[73] The second and third chapters of the novel are devoted to describing Catherine in detail:

> [S]he was not ugly; she had simply a plain, dull, gentle countenance . . . [and] though it is an awkward confession to make about one's heroine, I must add that she was something of a glutton. . . . Catherine was decidedly not clever. . . . She . . . developed a lively taste for dress . . . [but] I feel as if I ought to write it very small, her judgment in this matter was by no means infallible; it was liable to confusions and embarrassments.[74]

Although the reader is often tempted to conclude that such degrading depictions of Catherine are products of Austin's mind, the intriguing fact is that in the novel's early chapters, they belong to the narrative voice. As the story unfolds, the tenor of the narrator's comments about Catherine changes as she changes. Midway through the novel, his tone has shifted from one of frank condescension to one of surprised expectations: "Catherine meanwhile had made a discovery of a very different sort. . . . It was as if [an]other person, who was both herself and not herself, had suddenly sprung into being, inspiring her with a natural curiosity as to the performance of untested functions."[75] Here, the narrator appropriates and modifies the scientific and mathematical language previously dominated by men as a means to control and codify Catherine. By applying the traditionally rigid, formulae-defined concept of a function to Catherine while simultaneously pushing it into the nebulous realm of *untested* and therefore unquantifiable formulae, the narrator demonstrates Catherine's growth beyond predetermined definitions of "safe" existence. This description specifically sets itself against the former reference to Catherine's potential being "limited" by the functional equation of her mother. Here, Catherine is set into the realm of functions *without limits,* a newly emergent concept in the 1880s. Indeed, even as he repurposes historical trajectories to harness the cultural heft of contemporary obstetrics, James also builds the statistical and algebraic assessment of risk that undergirded Semmelweis's seminal studies into the narrative arc of *Washington Square.* In the early half of the nineteenth century, functions were indeed limited, conceptualized as simplistic renderings of relationships (much as Austin "limits" Catherine by her mother's capabilities in the beginning of the novel). However, by the 1870s, mathematicians were beginning to explore the potential for *irrational* numbers and *limitless* functions.[76] Statements such as these, casting Catherine in terms of new, innovative, and unlimited mathematical science, illustrate the narrator's changing attitudes about her during the course of the novel. These sentiments subtly continue to transform along with her own growing maturity, and by the conclusion, his statements about Catherine ring with notes of earnest admiration. This increasingly sympathetic narrative tone reaches its climax when she severs ties with her father's values once and for all. After her refusal to acquiesce to her father's request that she not marry Morris after his death, the narrator empathetically notes that while "Catherine's dignity was not aggressive . . . if you pushed far enough you could find it. Her father had pushed her very far."[77]

The narrator, like Catherine, has come full circle, beckoning readers to join him in recognizing the validity of and freedom promised by Catherine's final and paradoxical withdrawal—not from the world of community, but from a culture that hems in human interactions by speculative assessments of their utilitarian value and cost-benefit analyses of personal gain and risk. He notes that Catherine "knew she was obstinate, and it gave her a certain joy," once again avowing the righteousness of her actions and attitudes.[78] When Morris returns at the novel's conclusion for a final try at siphoning off a portion of Catherine's wealth for himself via marriage, she resists him firmly, not even asking him to sit down. The narrator wonders at "how old she had grown—how much she had lived!"[79] His altered attitude toward her is evident here and has clearly paralleled her own changing self-perceptions and path of personal growth. Catherine's change of heart is certainly discernible without the narrator. However, it is his changing allegiance during the plot that acts as *public* validation of her actions. Although originally aligned with Austin Sloper's condescending and devaluing views of her as an unprofitable byproduct of a failed business venture, the narrator's striking alliance with Catherine's self-determined, nonparticipatory views by the novel's conclusion—at a time when, after Austin's death, the views of the two can no longer be ambiguously conflated—therefore shows her acts in a new light which reveals them undeniably as emancipatory acts of resistance rather than defeatist movements of withdrawal. By changing allegiances in a manner that parallels Catherine's own personal growth, the narrative voice tags her resistant acts not as defeat in the form of spinsterhood, but as acts of reclaimed selfhood through nonparticipation—a refusal to engage in a worldview that casts interpersonal relationships as the sum of their counterpoised risks.

By the end of *Washington Square*, Catherine realizes that there is no possibility for *inter*action in a male world which fixates on self-assured safety from risk, and she finds meaningful existence through a complete refusal to participate in this mode of exchange and a cultivating of her own environment and social network. For Catherine, true *life* in terms of a meaningful and enriched existence can only come through nonparticipatory resistance to these prevailing social values. As Morris storms out of her home at the novel's conclusion, the now-supportive narrator concludes his account of Catherine's life by wryly draping his final description of her—a description of her independence and growth—in a statement that connotes mere spinsterism. For the reader who cannot, as Catherine has, break free from the predominant actuarial framework of human (especially female) value, the novel is a sad and anticlimactic one. For those who can keep up with the narrator and Catherine as they traipse bravely along the winding path to selfhood, the real meaning of the closing lines are apparent, as Catherine settles back in her chair, "for *life*, as it were."[80]

3

Separation and Suffocation

Tuberculosis, Etiological Uncertainty, and Female Friendship in Women's Fiction

Little Eliza . . . inherited, with her mother's beauty, her constitutional delicacy. . . . If she occasionally flitted for a moment into the world, its glare and uproar seemed almost to stun her gentle spirit.

—"Diary of a Late Physician," *Museum of Foreign Literature*, 1831

One poor young lady, a governess . . . attracts our attention. . . . alone and away from her own friends . . . coughing and expectorating in a sad helpless manner.

—"Brompton Consumption Hospital," *The Sunday at Home*, 1862

In passing, I may say we patients were very proud of our research laboratory.

—*The Cure of Consumption: A Message of Hope by One Who has Been Cured, Pall Mall*, 1903

The open-air sanatoria . . . [is a] successful . . . means of treating the disease. . . . The patient, breathing germ-free air . . . is found in a good many cases to recover. [But] restored to society, this patient may marry . . . [and] produce further offspring, who inherit their parent's tendency to tuberculous disease.

—W. C. Rivers, "Marriage and Tuberculosis," *Saturday Review*, 1902

"Sweet Dreams" and "Quiet Breathing":
The Changing Legacy of a Mystifying Killer

In 1978, Susan Sontag famously likened nineteenth-century social constructions of tuberculosis to twentieth-century cancer discourse. Her now-famous
monograph *Illness as Metaphor* opens by asserting that the "two diseases have
been spectacularly, and similarly, encumbered by the trappings of metaphor."[1]
Although *Illness as Metaphor* now stands on the far side of a nearly forty-year
chronological gap, Sontag's words ring true even today. As she explains:

> The fantasies inspired by TB in the last century, by cancer now,
> are responses to a disease thought to be intractable and capri-
> cious—that is, a disease not understood—in an era in which
> medicine's central premise is that all diseases can be cured.[2]

Like cancer today, tuberculosis seemed perplexingly indecipherable in the
nineteenth century, and it therefore developed an elusive and slippery set of
cultural meanings at odds with a society increasingly invested in the powers
of science and medicine to codify and combat disease. Even as the century
progressed toward the solidification of germ theory in the *fin-de-siècle,* tuberculosis remained a hazy concept, culturally unclarified by the identification
of its microbial pathogen. Unlike cholera, which was subject to productive
epidemiological analysis as early as the 1850s—well before germ theory would
come to fully dominate medical discourse—tuberculosis remained ethereal
and just outside the conceptual bounds of rational empiricism even into
the 1920s. This historical oddity is based partially on tuberculosis's rather
unique mode of transmission. If postpartum streptococcal infection spurred
intense germ theory debates because its quick incubation times and visible
symptoms led to its obvious, clearly observable communicability, tuberculosis
sparked wondering reflections about limits to the utility of germ theory due
to its ponderously slow incubation time, its low rate of infection, and its
often indeterminate symptomatology. This runs contrary to the view that
germ theory miraculously provided unequivocal truth once it arrived on the
world stage. In its own unique way, TB instead showcases how science and
society continually grapple with and influence each other.

Despite its veritable endemicity in the Victorian era, tuberculosis is
surprisingly difficult to contract. Only 25 percent of those exposed to the
mycobacterium will actually contract the disease (usually immunosuppressed
individuals), and of this number only a further 25 percent will ever expe-

rience an active, symptomatic infection, which may even then only show symptoms years after contraction.[3] Moreover, children are virtually immune to the disease, since the contagious vector cannot be inhaled deeply enough into their smaller respiratory tracts to proliferate effectively.[4] While rapidly spreading epidemics are difficult to control for their wildfire intensity, slowly germinating ones are epidemiological mysteries, with smoke trails difficult to see and nearly impossible to trace to their source. At first blush, it sounds reasonable that less-contagious illnesses are more easily controllable; in fact, they are just as uncontrollable for their elusiveness.

Blushes themselves are another reason for tuberculosis's etiological incomprehensibility. For a variety of reasons, the symptoms of tuberculosis were seen as aesthetically beautiful in the nineteenth century. As mentioned, TB is so difficult to contract that it generally impacts those who are already severely immunocompromised. And while dietary deficiencies, urban crowding, and frequent encounters with other diseases in the nineteenth century were indeed to blame for widespread susceptibility to the disease, the fevered flush brought on by tuberculosis was often seen as beautifying someone who had previously been sickly.[5] This "hectic" flush, shining eyes, pale skin, and thin waist came to represent an aesthetically appealing condition. As odd as this may seem to us today, compared against the emetic, hemorrhagic, and defecatory epidemics of the time, tuberculosis could indeed seem mild, peaceful, and even appealing to those living through it or watching their loved ones suffer from it. Additionally, because TB seemed to strike randomly, doctors came to believe that individuals had "differential susceptibility" to the disease.[6] Consequently, a mythos developed about TB "choosing" victims who were more fragile and delicate. This also lent to the perception that TB could be fashionable, as women in particular idealized what they saw as the nigh-angelic look of the pale, slender, rosy-cheeked consumptive. Indeed, as time went on, tubercular symptoms—frequently seen as they were in the population—came to define fashionable looks themselves. The "consumptive chic," as Carolyn Day has termed it, became in vogue and integral to the types of cosmetics and clothing marketed at the time.[7]

Though the height of the consumptive chic was the 1840s, the legacy of consumption as a beautiful disease persisted throughout the century in some degree or another. An 1884 treatise on the disease, for instance, describes the patients thusly:

The complexion is fair and frequently beautiful, as well as the features. The form, though delicate, is often graceful. The skin is

thin and of fine texture; the subcutaneous blue veins are numerous; showing very distinctly through the otherwise pearly white
integument. The pupils are usually spacious, and the eyeballs are
not only large, but prominent, the sclerotic showing a lustrous
whiteness. The eyelashes are long.[8]

Another defining aspect of tuberculosis allowed for the popularization of its
symptomatological aesthetics—because it could take decades for tuberculosis
to kill, it became in the nineteenth century like cancer is today: a disease
of life rather than an immediate cause of death. Partially because of this,
it has long been noted that Victorian society came to see TB as essentially
a disease of the self, rather than a disease of epidemics and society (like
cholera or puerperal fever).[9] As it became associated with a lifestyle rather
than a mode of death, those living with and around tuberculosis had the
opportunity to shape its lived ethos. If the "tubercular fashion" strikes us
as odd today, we need look no farther than the startling array of products
and apparel marked with breast cancer branding to see our own iteration
of this phenomenon—one that, again, demonstrates the veracity of Sontag's
claims regarding the similarities of cancer and TB.

Unlike so many other diseases of the nineteenth century that were
clear-cut in analysis, tuberculosis was marked by a triad of etiological con-
fusions: TB was unpredictable, it was slow, and it was quiet. The result of
these biostatistical facts was that, even after Robert Koch's discovery of the
tubercule bacillus in 1882, tuberculosis, unlike most other Victorian diseases,
remained a mysterious killer, striking seemingly random victims in mystifying
epidemiological paths.[10] The cultural meanings of consumption, then, fore-
shadowed twentieth-century battles with cancer; scrambles to identify risk
factors, mortality data, preventative methodologies, and cures saturated social
media of the period, much as pink ribbons and yellow wristbands do today.

While difficult to contract, consumption is even more difficult to trace
from person to person and killed an estimated 25 percent of Europeans and
Americans in the Victorian era—it was responsible for roughly 12 percent
of all deaths in Britain even into the early twentieth century. Because of
its paradoxical slow-burning prevalence, the disease was a discursive omnipresence throughout the century, though of course always subject to the
changing notions that science, along with doctors, patients, and loved ones,
could make of the illness.[11] As Rene and Jean Dubos, two historically classic
tuberculosis scientists and social historians, note:

Diseases manifest multiple personalities just as do living creatures and social institutions. The various moods which they display in different circumstances and at any given time reflect the dominant aspect of the relationship between the disease process and the life of man in society.[12]

More recently, Katherine Ott has put the matter this way:

The meaning of a disease evolves from the interrelationship of people, technology, medical doctrines, and state affairs. Illness is as dependent upon the palpable human experience of it as it is upon impersonal physiology and pathology.[13]

She continues that "there is neither a core 'tuberculosis,' constant over time, nor a smooth conceptual trajectory of the disease," as the societies that shape its meanings naturally change themselves.[14] As the previous chapter has shown, disease, particularly a disease whose trajectory is prevalent and publicized,

is a jumble of ideas that shifts among groups and over time. It is a cultural artifact configured in people's bodies, in medical doctrines, and in the physical material of illness. . . . Our confidence in the authority of science and its definitions tends to crowd out the ambiguities and untidy questions that looking at history often introduces.[15]

Under different guises—the disease was alternately called phthisis, consumption, and tuberculosis as the century progressed—it changed shape and meaning in fluid ways that did not necessarily mirror scientific progress but, rather, seemed to reflect man's relationship to microbial life.[16] A brief comparison may help make tuberculosis's unique role in literature clearer. Syphilis, which would come to be widely portrayed in literature later in the century (and which is the subject of the next chapter), had predictable, sexually transmitted pathways that created a niche market, as it were, for its fictional representation. Its uses in fiction were generally limited to discussions of marriage, sexuality, and sexual education. Conversely, tuberculosis's malleable and uncertain etiology opened it up to an array of uses in literature. The previous chapter illustrated the ways in which a disease of women gave sputtering starts and rampant publicity to germ theory debates; the next chapter, on syphilis, will demonstrate how, once it had gained widespread acceptance, germ theory impacted the policing and legislation of sexuality. In the present chapter, I will bring TB to bear upon the interim period as society struggled to make new meanings of individual diseases and the concept of disease more generally. Since tuberculosis was a disease whose contagious nature was debated even into the twentieth century, its inflection upon pushes for isolationist protections, and the countercultural movement of authors indicating the stifling nature of isolation and the importance of community, will be apparent as well.

Consumption in literature required more than just basic implementa- tion. Indeed, Byrne notes that consumption eluded categorical limitations and "could *not* be used as a simple signifier for social conflict and social responsibility."[17] Because of its unique biosocial amalgamation, TB, more than almost any other contemporary disease, exhibited changing manifestations over time—first as it was construed socially, and then in print and other public discourse. It demonstrates lucidly the fact that the truth claims of science are not magic bullets (to use scientific discourse prescient in the next chapter) that immediately alter social understandings of disease as they fall in line with the objective truth claims of science. Rather, both the scientific and the social shape one another in an ongoing double helix.

In the Romantic era, tuberculosis became a stand-in for Romantic sensitivities, a disease afflicting idealized and popularly beatified individuals. Affirming this idea both theoretically and chronologically, tuberculosis was viewed throughout the century—to greater or lesser degrees as the cultural milieu dictated—as an *inherited* constitutional debility. This iteration of the disease arguably prevailed most strongly in the mid-century, in the liminal space between miasma theory's and germ theory's respective predominances. As a disease of self, TB did not fit neatly into narratives of diseased spaces and unhealthy places, and yet (as mentioned previously) neither did it seem to obviously demonstrate clear communicability, as germ theory would have it. Its seemingly random or preferential (depending on which experts were discussing the matter) choice of victims lent itself, in this liminal conceptual space, to greater emphasis on familial constitutional tendencies.

It is worth taking a moment to address miasmatic environments and their perceived relevance to tuberculosis. Byrne rightly notes that no disease in "the hungry forties" could rightly escape examination through a sanitary lens that favored the then-predominant view that spaces could be intrinsically healthy or unhealthy.[18] However prominent miasmatic imagery was in this early period—and it certainly was—tuberculosis's epidemiological pathways did not apparently align readily with a purely environmental or sanitary understanding. Some of this is likely due to confirmation bias in a populace inclined to believe in the purity and cleanliness of the disease; however, as already discussed, the very nature of the disease itself also constituted this bias in a self-fulfilling feedback loop. Environment was therefore largely grafted onto prevailing theories about constitutional tendencies, and was seen oftentimes as a possible trigger (and in the later sanitorium movement a possible treatment), but never the sole cause of tuberculosis, which again sets the disease apart from other contemporary illnesses.[19] One physician's explanation illustrates the synthesis of these theoretical perspectives quite well: "For the occurrence of tuberculosis in any given case, two factors are necessary, the proper soil and the infectious agent. The first, which we call the predisposition, is either hereditary or acquired."[20]

Again, while diathesis theory necessarily undergirded both earlier and later iterations of the disease (it could be invoked to support both Romantic sensitivities and post-germ-theory imaginings of inherited immunodeficiencies), it appeared most strongly, and most independently as a concept, in the mid-century. Public discourse on the topic of inherited tendencies toward TB took many forms. The seed-and-soil metaphor developed in the mid-century period and was quite popular, hearkening to what we would describe today as an intrinsically weakened immune system more susceptible to the mycobacteria.[21] As one physician put it:

> It cannot be said of any disease proven to be dependent upon or associated with a specific infective particle that its presence or virulence is independent of person or surroundings. Even where the seed is not indigenous and the sower who goes forth to sow is unseen, yet if it falls by the beaten wayside, or where there is no depth of earth, in the unfriendly soil of a pure life or pure dwelling place it perishes as an invading army perishes without its commissariat.[22]

In 1859, George Meredith would cast the issue as one of aristocratic snobbery in the marriage market, as his protagonist Austin Feverel looks askance at the "consumptive daughter" of his friend, whom, though "there was something poetic about her," nevertheless he deems an unfit wife for his son due purely to her consumptive constitution.[23] As time shuffled onward toward germ theory's growing predominance, the diathesis model became the preferred mode of discussing the issue. That is, a person might inherit a constitutional tendency toward consumption that could be *triggered* by an unsettling life event which *activated* his or her constitutional weakness. Usually, this built upon the earlier Romantic model of emotional sensitivity. And so, in a time when medical treatments were uncertain, many physicians and laymen alike took the approach that those with an inherited weakness must be treated with extreme gentleness and surrounded by peaceful environments in order to avoid the dreaded activation of their natural, harbored proclivity to TB. Not just strong emotional experience, but also repressed passions were thought to be dangerous for their catalytic potential. Even into the twentieth century, decades after Robert Koch identified the mycobacteria responsible for the disease, eugenicists invoked this constitutional diathesis model, proclaiming that the disease could be eradicated if those with tubercular tendencies were barred from marriage. Tuberculosis was the nineteenth-century disease with the greatest ductility, and authors responded to it as such, pulling the strands of its metaphoric potential deftly in directions that suited their purposes.

In this chapter, I illustrate the different ends to which an array of female authors used the disease as a vessel by which to transmute their perspectives on bonds between women during a time when both tyrannical disease and hegemonic patriarchy loomed large. As Feldberg has noted, "examinations of differential susceptibility to TB" often specifically "probed the changing status of women" in its considerations.[24] By juxtaposing fictional productions of tuberculosis across the century (in roughly the same thirty-year segments shown in the epigraphs above), all of which—as I will show—package a single social question in their depiction of the disease, I isolate and investigate tuberculosis's tensile strength. Attuned to the remarkable metaphoric potential of disease, a host of female-authored novels—here, I have selected Charlotte Brontë's 1847 *Jane Eyre,* two mid-century sensation novels (Ellen Wood's *East Lynne* [1861] and Mary Elizabeth Braddon's *John Marchmont's Legacy* [1863]), and Ella Hepworth Dixon's 1894 *The Story of a Modern Woman*—use tuberculosis as a means of communicating their concerns about female friendship.[25] Each woman's use of tuberculosis exemplifies a vastly different embodiment of the disease; all of them, however, use the disease to demonstrate the necessity of female community in a patriarchal society. All of the novels use tuberculosis to resist the ideological isolation of women through the discourse of separate spheres and the language of domestic purity. In *Jane Eyre,* it serves to allow for a pure space where female homosociality can thrive. Particularly in the latter three novels, isolation from risk encounters—as seen in female friendships, which were seen to threaten the authority of patriarchal role in married women's lives—is flipped, and revealed not as protective, but as stifling and diseasing. The clear representational differences speak not only to changes in attitudes toward women or to the advances in scientific understanding that occurred during these decades but also to how the evolution of these two spheres circulated within and around one another in a mutually constitutive dance of socioscientific influence.

"Stifled Breath and Constricted Throat": Tuberculosis and Homosociality in *Jane Eyre*

Few can forget young Jane Eyre's first and virtually only childhood friend, Helen Burns, the kindhearted but much-maligned girl who befriends her at Lowood School. Although Jane expects to escape Gateshead's injustices at Lowood, she quickly finds herself disillusioned and cast as a reprobate at the charity school as well. During his first visit to the school, Mr. Brocklehurst publicly calls Jane a liar and forces her to stand upon a stool in the middle of the school room. Jane recounts her humiliation:

> I could not bear the shame of standing [there]. . . . What my sensations were no language can describe; but just as they all rose, stifling my breath and constricting my throat, a girl came up and passed me: in passing she lifted her eyes. What a strange light inspired them! What an extraordinary sensation that ray sent through me! How the new feeling bore me up! . . . What a smile! I remember it now, and I know that it was the effluence of fine intellect, of true courage.[26]

Although Jane and Helen are already acquainted at this point, their prior relationship had been somewhat cool, consisting primarily of Jane asking strings of childish questions of Helen, coupled with Helen's reluctantly proffered responses. When Jane makes eye contact with Helen from her stool, however, their relationship becomes forever marked by passion. Jane exclaims in her post-hoc narrative analysis that a "sensation" was "sent through her" by Helen's face. "*How* the new feeling bore me up," she continues, "*what* a smile," "*what* a strange light," and "*what* an extraordinary sensation": all these ejaculations probe potentialities of their by this point embodied relationship. Less memorable than Jane and Helen's homosocial friendship, however, are the precise contexts and manner of Helen's death, circumstances that embed the text firmly within early-century socioscientific discourse of tuberculosis. Brontë exploits the tropes of this discourse to imbue the girls' relationship with emotional and physical passion sustainable within the otherwise heteronormative bounds of *Jane Eyre*.

Jane describes her first spring at Lowood—the spring of Helen's death—as a thing of beauty, but she qualifies her claims:

> Have I not described a pleasant site for a dwelling, when I speak of it as bosomed in hill and wood, and rising from the verge of a stream? Assuredly, pleasant enough: but whether healthy or not is another question. That forest-dell, where Lowood lay, was the cradle of fog and fog-bred pestilence; which, quickening with the quickening of spring, crept into the Orphan Asylum, [and] breathed typhus through its crowded school-room.[27]

In introducing the typhus epidemic that will overtake Lowood, Brontë immediately works to separate this pestilential contagion from Helen's seemingly isolated case of consumption. The notion of "fog-bred pestilence" maps literally onto the early-century concept of miasmas (disease-spreading, poisonous airs that inhabited certain spaces, such as stuffy houses or rooms within homes). Even before the advent of germ theory and bacteriology, typhus was known to be a disease of overcrowding and famine, of poverty and filth, which often appeared in prisons or army camps. Jane goes on to explain that "semi-starvation and neglected colds had predisposed most of the pupils to receive infection" (thereby demarcating it from Helen's very separate disease) and later notes that a post-outbreak investigation into the school revealed that "the unhealthy nature of the site; the quantity and quality of the children's food; the brackish, fetid water used in its preparation; the pupils' wretched clothing and accommodation" all contributed to the epidemic.[28] All of these factors—threadbare clothing, stagnant drinking water, meager dietary accommodations—underscore the fact of Lowood's being an "orphan asylum" and therefore highlights the fact that "scourge" of typhus racing through its environs is the result of poverty and uncleanliness.[29]

Brontë does not vilify the young victims for their impoverished condition; however, the specific identification of the pathogen as typhus (a rare detail in early-century novels where vaguely identified "fevers" and "chills" were explanation enough) pointedly grounds this outbreak in class concerns. Brontë also clearly tags the epidemic as highly infectious, in spite of the paradoxical early reference to a miasmatic environment. Jane calls Lowood a "seat of contagion," a phrase clearly grounded in germ theory, remarking that the housekeeper was "driven away by the fear of infection."[30] In spite of this sense of communicability, miasma discourse nevertheless pervades her preceding and subsequent descriptions of the illness, intertwining itself with rhetoric of germs and infection. Jane explains that doctors attended the Lowood patients but to little avail, "the drug and the pastille striving vainly to overcome the effluvia of mortality," "effluvia" being perhaps one of the most predominant buzzwords of miasma theory.[31] This word, situated between two sentences describing the infectious principle of the epidemic, binds miasmatic and contagious elements together in Jane's descriptions of the outbreak. Thus, typhus in *Jane Eyre* is construed as a disease bred by the unhealthy, fog-laden air, then cultivated in the children's weakened and dirty bodies, and finally spread among them after they become contagious. The epidemic at Lowood, then, is one of sepsis- *and* miasma-based contagion, rendering visible the multimodal avenues of contaminated contact. These trails of contact bring to mind Priscilla Wald's famous analysis of epidemiology, in which she argues that "disease emergence dramatizes the dilemma that inspires the most basic of human narratives: the necessity and danger of human contact."[32] Of course, Jane never contracts the highly contagious typhus. Nor does Helen, although she dies during the outbreak. Helen, Jane's most cherished and highly idealized friend, dies instead of tuberculosis, and her decline is depicted with the standard romantic tropes that surrounded consumption in the early parts of the century.

In *Consumption and Literature: The Making of a Romantic Disease*, Clark Lawlor notes that "in the Romantic formulation, consumption was aestheticized in a positive manner as a sign of passion, spirituality and genius."[33] In fact, tuberculosis was often viewed as a constitutional inability to flourish amid the hectic, immoral, and materialistic world. As Byrne has shown, in many cases it "function[ed] as a cultural metaphor for this kind of economic process, for [its] gradual wasting and using up of the body's resources of flesh and strength clearly made it a perfect signifier for the dangers of excess and consumerism."[34] Indeed, the conceptualization of consumption as the "death warrant" for those who were "unable to withstand contact with the crude world" preceded the death of John Keats but was also greatly reinforced by it.[35] Although Keats may have been the "archetyp[e] of consumptive geni[us]," Lawlor explains, even before the Romantic era, poets were considered highly susceptible to tuberculosis because they were endowed with "fine nerves, an enhanced sensibility to the point of excessive suffering when in contact with the rough, 'insensible' world."[36] And, although Gaskell and Dickens would poignantly go on to portray tubercular deaths in their industrial novels as a horrific scourge of the working class, tuberculosis was in many ways a disease whose connotative categorization was imbued with aspirational class consciousness in the first half of the century. Lawlor notes that "the rise of the idea of the Romantic poet helped to push consumption to prime position in the hierarchy of alluring diseases. Aspiring lower-class young men might rise to fame via possession of a disease which authenticated one's poetic credentials."[37] For women in particular, "consumption was a beautiful disease; it was spiritual and consoling; and it was also still a malady of desire and love."[38] Consumptives, then, in the early parts of the nineteenth century, were seen as constitutionally too perfect for this world, marred and scarred by it, then finally departing from it peacefully in angelic repose that, in fiction, often elided the horrifying realities concomitant with slow pulmonary failure.

Helen Burns, whose name hearkens to Romantic poet Robert Burns in an almost heavy-handed manner, is given one of the most quintessentially romanticized tubercular deaths in all of Victorian literature, second perhaps only to Little Eva's in *Uncle Tom's Cabin*. During this period in the literary imaginary, death from pulmonary tuberculosis did not merely afflict the pure and delicate, it also bestowed upon these patients a delicate, pure death. Sputum and expectoration, which were of course part and parcel of tuberculosis, never appear in early-century death scenes. Instead, tubercular deaths in fiction and the popular press during this period are portrayed as peaceful, slow, and generally beautiful, providing the main character (who is, as a matter of course, fittingly pure as well) enough time to monologue about charity, love, and the afterlife. True to form, Helen's deathbed is adorned with "white curtains" indicative of her purity, even amid the pestilence that scourges the rest of Lowood.[39] She is also separated physically from the common sickroom, sequestered in both moral and aseptic purity—and of course from the class considerations that weigh down the rest of the pupils in messy, earthly problems such as poverty and hunger. Helen's diseased body is tropologically beautiful as well, for although Jane initially "recoil[s] at the dread of seeing a corpse" when she visits Helen, she is instantly reassured by Helen's countenance, "pale, wasted, but still composed" and "little changed."[40] Her beautifully wasted body is a typical fictive portrayal of tubercular death in this period, particularly in regard to female death from consumption. None of the Kristevan horrors of mortality accompany consumptive death in the first half of the century—ideologically speaking, that is. Jane is, in fact, so much encouraged by Helen's mien that she recalls thinking, "She is not going to die; they are mistaken: she could not speak and look so calmly if she were."[41] Indeed, in spite of her imminent death, Helen speaks piously and calmly of her own demise (in accord with the typical ficto-tubercular protocol of the time), telling Jane that she is going to her "long home," and responding to Jane's grief by saying,

> I am very happy, Jane. And when you hear that I am dead, you must be sure and not grieve: there is nothing to grieve about. We must all die one day, and the illness which is removing me is not painful; it is gentle and gradual: my mind is at rest. . . . By dying young, I shall escape great sufferings. . . . I am going to God. . . . I count the hours till that eventful one arrives which shall restore me to him, reveal him to me.[42]

As they talk, Jane snuggles up to Helen's body under a quilt, and the two hold one another affectionately while Jane occasionally kisses her friend, free from any fear of contagion in this moment of spiritual connection. Just before the two drift off to sleep, a repose during which Helen will die, she reassures Jane once more: "How comfortable I am! That last fit of coughing has tired me a little; I feel as if I could sleep."[43]

Helen's demise is perhaps the quintessential Romantic representation of death by tuberculosis in fiction. By meticulously aligning her description of Helen's decline with all the markers of celestial purity so typical of romanticized portrayals of consumption in this period, Brontë subtly uses this literary configuration to situate Helen and Jane's relationship in a pure space above moral reproach and outside of the grip of typical human concerns (such as poverty, contagion, hunger, cold, or thirst). Importantly, at a time prior to germ theory's tightening vise grip on Victorian culture, Brontë selectively parses out her use of socioscientific discourse in order to demarcate Helen's ethereal illness from Lowood's fleshy one, all for the paradoxical end (as we will see) of successfully *embodying* Jane and Helen's relationship. To successfully represent their highly embodied interactions, that is, Brontë must rather counterintuitively carve out an irreproachable moral environment for the two which, because of Helen's consumption, can appear untainted by any erotic charge despite its marked physicality. The moral purity of those touched with consumption was standard in tuberculosis discourse up through the first half of the century; thus, contemporary readers would have been particularly attuned to Helen's purity, and, by association, Jane's. More to the point, the emphasis in the text on the contagious scourge of typhus that is raging through Lowood—described in the novel as its source of "infection," "contagion," and rampant "mortality"—juxtaposed with Helen's consumption, which places her in a *cordon sanitaire,* allows Jane and Helen to engage in what would otherwise be seen as a risk encounter and embody their relationship in caresses and kisses.[44] Jane describes her journey to Helen's room, explaining that the acrid "odour of camphor and burnt vinegar" warned her away from the rooms of typhus patients while leading her to the fresher air, as it were, of Helen's sickroom.[45] The space occupied by Helen is neither infectious nor pervaded with foul miasmas, but, rather, a room of their own that allows for both physical intimacy and imaginative and spiritual inspiration. Within this impeccable moral space, Brontë has given herself room to traverse the full potential of female homosociality, as Jane and Helen clutch one another in bed, caressing and kissing during one of the most passionate scenes of the novel, as well as in the range of literature that I will cover in this book.

However, while Helen's last moments are imbued with many of the tropes of Romantic consumption, her actual death and its aftermath are glossed over. Death in nineteenth-century fiction typically offers a moment of pause wherein the author, via an omniscient, third-person narrator, offers any number of religious or existential reflections, particularly if the deceased is allied with the protagonist. Jane, however, reflects only momentarily on Helen's death:

> A day or two afterwards I learned that Miss Temple, on returning to her own room at dawn, had found me laid in a little crib; my face against Helen Burn's shoulder, my arms around her neck. I was asleep, and Helen was—dead. Her grave is in Brocklebridge churchyard; for fifteen years after her death it was only covered by a grassy mound; but now a grey marble tablet marks the spot, inscribed with her name, and the word "Resurgam."[46]

For being otherwise so representative of the Romantic tubercular decline, Helen's actual death is nearly completely elided, making it quite the opposite, for instance, of Little Eva's equally archetypal tubercular death, after which the narrator devotes nearly an entire chapter to reflection upon "the frail seed of that bright, immortal form" and to lament, "there is no death to such as thou, dear Eva!"[47]

Cloaked in the guise of mere trope-treading, Brontë's descriptions of consumption deftly incorporate female intimacy that at times verges on the

erotic; she then suddenly shores up her descriptions and changes the subject. Brontë's meticulous adherence to the tropes of consumption only calls
attention to these moments of tropic deviation. There is in her diversions an
important expression of passion a shade too intense to fit perfectly within
these tropological strictures, of nonchalance slightly too showy to be taken at
face value. Because tuberculosis was often ideologically construed as a disease
of repression and passion, Helen's consumptive death textually points even
more insistently toward the risky encounter of the homosocial or homoerotic
nature of her relationship with Jane. Cleverly, the purity conferred upon
Helen by her consumption situates her (and Jane by association) beyond
the pale of moral reproach while, conveniently, her inevitable death allows
Jane to maintain the veracity of these homosocial bonds with impunity
while integrating herself within the heteronormative marriage necessary for
a "successful" conclusion to her *bildungsroman*. Brontë cleverly subverts
tubercular tropes, therefore, in her description of Helen and Jane's sensual
relationship in order to showcase the productive potential of homosocial
female bonds and spaces that countenance them. Indeed, Mary Armstrong
claims similarly that this scene "spin[s] out Jane's desire along the axis of
Helen's erotic abilities and then shut[s] that trajectory down" as a way of
"open[ing] up female homoerotics and then compress[ing] them below the
heteroerotic surface. . . . These desires further establish that gender is in fact
not the organizing factor for such pleasures."[48] Although the novel resolves
within a heteronormative framework, this early sexual subversion serves as
an instance of embedded resistance to it in that it both questions the value
of its own heteronormative ending and destabilizes the worth of gendered
binaries as structuring paradigms in society.

In this guise, Helen's narrative strand stretches unto the novel's concluding pages. The last direct reference to Helen in the novel is Jane's statement
in these early chapters that her grave went unmarked for "fifteen years"; after
mentioning the now-extant headstone's inscription, "resurgam," she abruptly
changes the subject and advances the narrative forward in time another eight
years.[49] This casual mention of a fifteen-year gap between Helen's death
and provision of a tombstone is buried passingly (like Helen) in the early
chapters of the novel. However, this chronological fast-forward, as it were,
neatly settles at the novel's conclusion just after Jane and Rochester's marriage—which occurs precisely fifteen years after Helen's death. Thus, Helen's
narrative strain is coyly strung along throughout the entirety of Brontë's
heteronormative Gothic romance and woven into the warf of its ending. It is
clearly Jane, lately become an heiress, who has used her independent wealth

to commemorate her most meaningful relationship, even as she narrates the conclusion of a story ostensibly about a different relationship altogether. Like the epitaph that seemingly concludes her story, Helen "rises again" at the novel's conclusion through the presentist gesture that Jane includes in the novel's early pages that signals her long-standing and continued investment in their relationship. While Jane may have externally obeyed the dictates of heteronormativity in her marriage to Rochester, her anachronistic reference to Helen, which situates a reference to her old friend precisely at the point of this nuptial event, subtly insists upon attendance to the powerful effects that homosocial relationships have made in Jane's life. As Armstrong points out, *Jane Eyre* depicts "transgressive female homoerotic possibilities which are frequent and unstable, yet seamlessly woven into one of the most well-known heterosexual romance stories in English literature."[50] Brontë's descriptions of Jane and Helen clasping one another fervently (and rather furtively) coalesce with romantic tubercular portraits. They also extrapolate beyond themselves, questioning the potential of the passionate, embodied individuals they mythologize; Brontë probes the depths of this potential, situated as she was just short of the precipice of an era wherein any and all bonds between women would come under scrutiny.

"Fighting for Breath": Female Rivalry in *East Lynne*

As the century progressed, the potential for productive friendships between women came to be viewed with increasing skepticism. In the first quarter of the century, whimsical poems lauding female friendships appeared occasionally in newspapers (an 1813 poem titled "Female Friendship" opens with the claim that "joy cannot claim a purer bliss, / . . . than female friendship's meeting kiss," for instance).[51] New Woman treatises at the *fin-de-siècle* would later speak to the important power of female solidarity. Conversely, the mid-century saw a barrage of texts that argued against the possibility or, at least, the value of female friendships, largely insofar as they diverted virile energy away from heterosexual marital relations. To cite just one periodical essay, "Women's Friendships" (published at least three times in 1866), asserts that female relationships are comprised of a "much more violent feeling than male friendship. It is something much more like love . . . [and] actually clashes in some cases with the love of married life, which male friendship distinctly does not."[52] Its author concludes: "We suspect that the relations of women to one another . . . are all grounded on the weaker parts of their characters, and are likely . . . to strengthen their weaknesses, instead of communicating any better and stronger elements."[53]

Published fourteen years after *Jane Eyre* and in this environment averse to female friendship, Ellen Wood's wildly popular sensation novel *East Lynne* constructs a hegemonically palatable ideology that inhibits the development of female-female relationships. Like *Jane Eyre*, however, while *East Lynne* seemingly embeds itself in discourse of the day which would deny women's bonds, its narrative trajectory serves in fact to warn against a society in which women can only exist as rivals to one another—and this subversive narrative undercurrent exists solely in its use of tubercular tropes. Wood's novel, I argue, works to suggest the problems of casting women in the ideological imaginary as nothing more than embodied risk encounters—both to themselves and others. To do so, Wood uses tuberculosis—to which *East Lynne*'s protagonist, Isabel Vane, eventually succumbs—as a means by which to demonstrate her sense of the importance of female friendships. As I will show, Isabel Vane, who is less obviously showcased as a consumptive than Helen Burns, is nevertheless tagged early on in the novel as the recipient of a dormant tubercular constitution activated by a world in which her only productive relationships are intended to be with men, and in which her only relationships with women are characterized by obsessive jealousy and suspicion. Like that of Helen, Isabel's eventual death from tuberculosis similarly allows Wood to craft a space of redemption and freedom for Isabel, in spite of her sexual transgressions that make up much of the novel's plot. Thus, Isabel's consumptive legacy allows Wood, like Brontë before her, to subtly package subversive claims about women's relationships to one another into an otherwise inoffensive novel that purportedly upholds the moral status quo, developing earlier iterations of female-authored literature on this subject.

East Lynne is the story of the young and beautiful Lady Isabel Vane, who is left destitute after the death of her profligate father, the late Lord Mount Severn. Forced to live in a state of dependency with relatives, she quickly accepts a marriage proposal from the unfailingly (and somewhat unrealistically) righteous, moral, and clear-sighted Archibald Carlyle. Though she has no feelings for Archibald, Isabel agrees to the marriage because it guarantees her financial security. While she is relatively satisfied with her marriage, she is plagued by her overbearing and condescending sister-in-law, Cornelia Carlyle, who comes to live with them, as well as by her own misguided suspicions that her husband is having an affair with a neighbor, Barbara Hare. Isabel's discontent is compounded by the fact that she falls ill after she begins bearing children—what is initially thought to be a common postpartum infection transforms within lines into tuberculosis during a fit of jealousy. Fueled by her suspicions of her husband's infidelity, she eventually abandons her marriage for a more passionate relationship with the rakish Francis Levison, who (as rakes are wont to do) later abandons her. After a disfiguring train wreck, she returns to her marital home in disguise as a governess, only to discover that Archibald (who has by this time obtained a divorce) has married Barbara. Isabel now for the first time falls in love with Archibald, but it is much too late, and she spends the final portions of the novel raising her own children as a stranger under the roof of her former marital home, keeping her identity a secret until her tubercular death under their roof.

Isabel's vaguely defined postpartum illness is readily identifiable, as descriptions of it are laden with the contemporary hallmarks of tuberculosis. She is described as having "pallid cheeks" that "burn . . . with a red hectic glow," as well as "eyes [that] glisten . . . with fever."[54] These three elements—unnatural pallor, "hectic" complexion, and shining, febrile eyes—are the three most common descriptors of tuberculosis in Victorian fiction. They are so common that they nearly always function as metonyms for the disease; "tuberculosis" and "consumption" need not be specifically mentioned (although they are in *East Lynne*). The word *hectic* is used, in fact, in almost no other contexts in Victorian writing. Although her immediately postpartum condition is described in terms similar to the very common "childbed" or puerperal fever (being identified solely as a fever and weakness developed after parturition), she never quite recovers from this weakness, and it transforms into a readily identifiable case of tuberculosis. Moreover, the disease is fueled by her continued jealousy of Barbara Hare, for her "pallid" coloring and "hectic" cheeks only emerge after she overhears a conversation outside of her sickroom regarding Barbara Hare's continued love for her husband, who a maid speculates will marry Archibald if Isabel dies from her illness.

As will become clear, Isabel's tubercular decline is intimately bound up with the social protocols restricting her positive interactions with women. For instance, there are two sexually desirable men in the story—Archibald and Francis—and all the women in the story hover in perpetual covetous orbit around them: Isabel grapples with her distant relative and successor to her revoked title, Lady Emma Mount Severn over Francis's attentions; Barbara and Isabel are consistently pitted against one another as rivals for Archibald's attentions, and even Cornelia and Isabel compete for mastery of Archibald's domestic affairs. Again and again, *East Lynne* depicts acts of female animosity, emotional aggression, and even violence toward other women. In fact, in spite of the "sensational" elements of the novel, which, typically, circulate around heterosexual relationships, the attention of the reader and most of the action focus on the interactions of these volatile women who hover in the background of nearly every event.

The most explicit instance of such violence occurs when Isabel is struck by Emma, who is "repellent" and "insolently patronizing" and who hates her.[55] The attack takes place on an evening when Emma accuses Isabel of flirting with Levison, Emma's cousin and the object of her affections. At this point, the narrator—always didactic and moralizing (and often apparently misogynistic)—steps in boldly, warning the reader of the consequences "when women, liable to intemperate fits of passion, give reins to them," for "they neither know nor care what they say."[56] After this finger-wagging digression, Isabel responds in kind, remarking haughtily that she prefers to "leave [flirting] . . . to married women," thereby implicating Emma as the subject of her own insulting accusation.[57] Emma is livid:

> The home truth told on her ladyship. She turned white with rage, forgot her manners, and, raising her right hand, struck Isabel a stinging blow upon the left cheek. Confused and terrified, Isabel stood in pain, and before she could speak or act, my lady's left hand was raised to the other cheek, and a blow left on that. Lady Isabel shivered as with a sudden chill, and cried out, a sharp, quick cry; covered her outraged face and sank down upon the dressing chair.[58]

The violence makes the episode unforgettable; the reader, like Isabel, remains stunned for some time.

While Emma's blows constitute the only female-female *physical* violence, the novel is replete with other representations of female animosity toward women. For example, Isabel's "jealous eyes" become a structuring motif in the text, as they watch Barbara from various vantage points. They watch from Isabel's "dressing-room window" as Barbara and Archibald "stroll . . . down the park, deep in . . . [conversation] and quite unconscious" of her spiteful stares.[59] Later, Barbara calls upon Archibald at East Lynne; he "accompanie[s] her as far as the park gates," and the two are "absorbed in earnest converse."[60] "Lady Isabel's jealous eyes saw that," the narrator succinctly informs the reader.[61] When Barbara receives a letter from her fugitive brother, she brings it to Archibald for his opinion, and he reads it with her, "neither of them thinking that Lady Isabel's jealous eyes" are surveying their actions.[62] Even when Isabel returns in disguise as the family's governess, her "jealous eyes . . . turn . . . upon them" as they kiss "fondly" in the drawing-room.[63] As previously mentioned, it is initially Isabel's frantic jealousy of Barbara that converts her vague "fever and weakness" into the characteristic consumptive "hectic," for it is not until she overhears a servant predicting that "Barbara, as sure as fate, would step into [Isabel's] shoes" in the event of her death, that the narrator first describes Isabel's fever as marked by the tubercular triad of "pallid cheeks," a "hectic glow," and "glisten[ing]" eyes.[64]

Barbara's reciprocal jealousy of Isabel's power over Archibald is depicted in similar terms. Her "covetous eyes" stare greedily at Isabel during church, and she must "compel . . . her voice to calmness" in even inquiring about Isabel.[65] Another incident occurs after Archibald and Isabel's marriage. Barbara had visited the couple at East Lynne, and Archibald walked her home. The "evident happiness" of the couple, the narrator explains, stirs in Barbara "a state of nervous excitement when temper, tongue, and imagination fly off at a mad tangent," at which point she attempts to confess her love for him.[66] But her intense jealousy renders her senseless, and before she can begin to express her feelings, she is overcome by a bout of "passion, temper, wrongs, and nervousness, all boiling over together."[67]

The most frequently depicted rivalry between women in *East Lynne* is that between the increasingly fading, consumptive Isabel and her sister-in-law, Cornelia, whose oppressive presence weighs on Isabel. From the moment Archibald tells his sister of his intended marriage, he suspects "that his sister would be bitter at the prospect."[68] "Of all women," the narrator adds, "the most objectionable to her would be Lady Isabel, for Miss Carlyle looked to the useful, and had neither sympathy nor admiration for the beautiful."[69] Although the malice between Cornelia and Isabel never escalates to a physical level, Cornelia's is perhaps the most palpably structuring malice in the entire novel. The narrator explicitly states that:

> Isabel would have been altogether happy but for Miss Carlyle;
> that lady still inflicted her presence upon East Lynne, and made
> it the bane of its household. She deferred outwardly to Lady
> Isabel as the mistress; but the real mistress was herself. Isabel
> was little more than an automaton. Her impulses were checked,
> her wishes frustrated, her actions tacitly condemned by the
> imperiously-willed Miss Carlyle.[70]

Though Tess Cosslett has noted that female rivalries are often transformed into fruitful friendships in Victorian fiction, *East Lynne* stops far short of this dynamic.[71] For instance, Isabel and Emma never reconcile. Barbara and Isabel, too, go on hating each other to the end and speak to each other on only a few occasions. However, the absence of female friendship in this novel is no mere absence. Rather, this void of female camaraderie becomes such a palpable presence of violent malice that it virtually structures the novel itself in place of the heterosexual relationships that typically structure sensation novels.[72] Certainly, Isabel's obsessively jealous thoughts regarding the affair she supposes her husband is carrying on with Barbara preoccupy the reader more than does her husband's day-to-day office business, or even the novel's rather slapdash murder mystery involving Barbara's brother. Thus, these moments of aggression highlight early on the structuring power of *female* relationships even as they purport to deny their value. Moreover, Archibald's overwrought perfection serves to indicate that male worth is of no consequence; good or bad though the husband may be, women's relationships are both more powerful and more important—and their repression has dire consequences. Since the romanticized ideals of tuberculosis were still pervasive at mid-century, the notion that consumption was a disease of repressed passions still had much popular sway. Wood deftly intertwines her critique of negated female relationships with tubercular discourse when she closes the chapter chronicling the transformation of Isabel's postpartum fever into full-blown tuberculosis with a narrative interjection that expounds upon jealousy between women in place of unity: "There was never a passion in this world—there never will be one—so fantastic, so delusive, so powerful as jealousy."[73]

Representation of women's repressed emotions is seen throughout *East Lynne*. In the novel's first chapter, when Isabel's father relates his history to Archibald, he notes that Isabel's mother died of consumption, which he believes was brought on by her despair in believing she caused her own father's death by eloping with her husband.[74] Although Lord Mount Severn seems puzzled, noting that "consumption never had been in her family," Wood's invocation of the disease in this context grows out of the notion of the consumptive diathesis that was prevalent in Victorian discourse.[75] As mentioned earlier, tuberculosis was often seen as a disease of repressed passions, frequently unrequited love. As an 1860 article on consumption explains: "nothing is more common than for the symptoms of consumption to . . . [be] brought on by deep and long-continued mental affliction."[76]

The early-century faith in the constitutional weakness showcased by consumptives had by the mid-century paired with notions of degenerate heredity to create a view of tuberculosis that continued to view the disease as a constitutional weakness, but, more importantly, as an inherited weakness.[77] Victorians thus believed that one inherited a tendency to develop consumption, rather than the disease itself. According to mid-century conceptualizations particularly, consumptive patients inherited a constitutional inability to withstand extreme emotional stress or repressed desires, an inheritance that might or might not surface as fatal consumption, depending on one's environment. As I have already mentioned, this is precisely what happens to Isabel. Her fairly common postpartum illness converts into active tuberculosis in direct response to overhearing a conversation about her rival.

Moreover, since the consumptive nature of Isabel's mother is mentioned in the novel's first chapter, the contemporary reader would have been immediately clued in to Isabel's ineluctable inherited inability to withstand the strain and stifled emotions she is forced to endure. There are, in fact, a number of clues suggesting Isabel's constitutional weakness in tropological terms that are clearly indicative of tuberculosis. The narrator describes her as "more timid and sensitive by nature than many would believe or can imagine . . . Isabel was unfit to battle with the world."[78] When Archibald first suggests to Isabel that his domineering sister Cornelia come to live with them after their marriage, the narrator signals Isabel's displeasure: "Isabel's heart sank within her at the idea of that stern Miss Corny, mounted over her as resident guard."[79] The narrator takes care to note, however, that Isabel makes no verbal objection to this plan, explaining that "refined and sensitive" as she was, "almost painfully considerate of the feelings of others, she raised no objection."[80] Isabel's "almost painful" empathy for others sets her up to fall victim to death and disease in the face of isolation, given the medical cosmologies of the day. Indeed, in the chapter describing Cornelia's effect upon Isabel's marital home (aptly titled) "Death or Life," the narrator goes on to reiterate Isabel's impending ruin in her state of isolation and as the target of antipathy: "Poor Isabel, with her refined manners and her timid and sensitive temperament, had no chance against the strong-minded woman, and she was in a state of galling subjection in her own house."[81] Isabel's responses to emotional stress are often expressed in terms of pulmonary distress. After her father's death early in the novel, for instance, Isabel learns not only that is she impoverished but also that her father died without paying an array of tradesmen, who have confronted her asking for payments she cannot make; as she speaks to the men in helpless apology, "her breath was labored with the excess of her tribulation."[82] Her breathing is once again described as "very labored" when she thanks Archibald for his help in dealing with the men and other dilemmas left behind by her father.[83]

In a novel in which female friendships are so threatening to patriarchal authority that their very possibility is repressed throughout the entire novel, it is Isabel's consumptive constitution that renders her incapable of tolerating her environment, which allows her no points of connection with other women. This deep-seated inability to tolerate stifled emotions leads directly to her flight from her husband's home. Cast against a contemporaneous understanding of disease and degeneracy, Isabel's dependence on her husband, and even her economically motivated marriage, suggests that her situation in an environment where female camaraderie is checked catalyzes her degeneracy and thus her consumption. Ann Cvetkovich notes further that "repression rather than oppression is the focus of the novel's drama; women whose feelings are generated by their structural position bear the additional burden of being forced to hide those feelings, stay silent, and put up with their lot in life."[84] Thus, considering the decisive nature with which the text repeatedly resists the possibility for female camaraderie, and given the prevalence of the notion that tuberculosis resulted from repressed or stifled emotions, Isabel's death represents not so much her punishment for sexual transgression as the fatal result of a life spent in isolation from anyone in whom she could truly confide. Although she dies, as is the common fate of sexually independent Victorian novel heroines, her consumptive constitution suggests her inherited inability to withstand the stifled world of female relationships into which she was born, and her romanticized tubercular death at the novel's conclusion reiterates her innocence.

Although the death of a fallen woman is a trope used long before the nineteenth century, it took on new and renewed significance in the mid-Victorian period. Isabel's eventual consumptive death is necessitated not simply because of her fallenness, but because her fallenness took on new and threatening implications in light of the popular scientific discourse of the day. Following the publication of *On the Origin of Species* (1859), Victorian society began to extrapolate beyond evolution to questions of *de*volution. If species could evolve into more and more perfect forms, Victorians worried, could they not also devolve into less perfected forms? Thus began a great and concerted effort to preserve the nature of man in its cultured state. Paradoxically, although evolution was first compellingly postulated by Darwin, concomitant fears of degeneration relied on earlier Lamarckian notions of acquired characteristics, which enabled blending notions of inheritance and genetic evolution with an ideological component that accounted for environment and lifestyle.[85] Much as Brontë's early-century depiction of consumption could seamlessly blend miasma discourse and the rhetoric of infection, so too did Darwinian and Lamarckian ideas intertwine in the mid-century into what became essentially eugenicist arguments regarding the contamination of bloodlines with congenital weaknesses. Acts such as Isabel's sexual transgression, then, seemed to herald the beginning of a descent back to a primal state. Additionally, although tuberculosis itself was not universally considered contagious in this mid-century period, its degenerative potential—encapsulated in its inheritable constitutional pro-clivities—were. Isabel, then, is a double-degenerate, both in her external actions and her inherent consumptive constitution. It would seem that her death is doubly mandated.

Of course, the anxiety about what to do textually with a sexually active woman (the answer to which often, in Victorian fiction, seemed to be to throw her into the Thames) is nothing new. Wood, however, deftly uses tuberculosis to solve an old authorial problem—she has Isabel, remarkably, survive a grisly train wreck, and then, just when all well-read Victorians would anticipate her dramatic death, Wood allows her to return home to die a peaceful death of slow, wasting consumption—a death, as we have seen, usually reserved for only the most pure of characters. The message of this tragically typical fallen woman story seems clear at first blush—transgression of the patriarchal norms results in ruin and death. Like Brontë, however, Wood bedecks her heroine and her journey with the discourse regarding the romantic "good death" of tuberculosis, in the process becoming not a stereotypically sentimental female novelist but, rather, an author boldly critiquing a society that denies women affirming bonds with one another.[86] Anne-Marie Beller supports such a reading, noting that "for Wood, death cannot be considered a punishment in any *straightforward* way."[87] "Rather," she asserts, "female death and disease is, for Wood, "the site at which con-flicting constructions of femininity collide and are negotiated."[88]

Read in light of this socioscientific context, Isabel's death takes on radical implications. The determinacy suggested by the contemporary under-standing of consumption as hereditary mitigates Isabel's culpability in her own actions and highlights her purity rather than her degeneracy. Her death, rather than being conventionally punitive, allows Wood to mount a harsh critique of the society that instituted the ideological system that catalyzed her death in the first place. The romantic tropes surrounding consumption serve to subtly vindicate her textually; Isabel dies "quite peacefully," evinc-ing, even in the last stages of severe pulmonary disease, only a moment of "slight struggle . . . a fighting for breath."[89] By the time of her passing, it is clear that Isabel has been "fighting for breath" throughout the whole novel, her inspiration oppressed by a society that has isolated her from any meaningful contact with other women. Ultimately, in providing Isabel with the "good" consumptive death, the text simultaneously mitigates her culpability and places the blame for her death on an ideological system that isolates women from one another.

Thus, although these two novels incorporate different representations of female friendship, depictions tightly intertwined with evolving scientific discourse, both use this discourse to carve out a space for female imagination and connection. In *Jane Eyre*, Helen and Jane can simply be together in privacy and with passion, in a space sequestered for them away from the grit and grime of more "common" illnesses, and therefore metaphorically away from hegemonic norms. In *East Lynne*, although Isabel dies without ever finding this sort of companionship, she nevertheless sidesteps the traditional textual consequence for female sexual agency and is granted a peaceful and easy death that marks her continued purity in spite of the hegemonic norms that stifle her throughout the novel. Both Jane and Isabel are able to deftly weave in and around these normative standards, fulfilling its mandates when necessary, but simultaneously finding freedom through adherence to these mandates (in plot and in trope) to breathe freely, and according to their own desires.

"An Air of Hopeless Indifference": Female Apathy in *John Marchmont's Legacy*

Mary Elizabeth Braddon, who began writing fiction about the same time as Wood, used tuberculosis to similar purpose in her 1863 novel, *John Marchmont's Legacy*. In fact, this novel might be read as a hyperbolic rendering of the themes just elucidated in *East Lynne*. The plot, like that of many sensation novels, hinges on fortunes and finance. The book opens with an encounter between the titular John Marchmont and an ex-pupil, Edward Arundel. During their reunion, Marchmont expresses concern that he may inherit his legendary fortune (for which he is third in line) and subsequently die young. In this event, he explains to Edward, his fortune would then be left to his unprotected daughter, Mary, whom he fears would be no match for her malicious, fortune-hungry relatives. *John Marchmont's Legacy* opens, then, with a straightforward discussion of the problems surrounding John Marchmont's financial legacy. However, the novel is equally about his *constitutional* legacy, for even before John's fortune is mentioned, the reader is introduced to his consumptive cough. Just as Jane first encounters Helen when she hears "the sound of a cough close behind" her, the narrator first metonymically introduces John Marchmont by *his* "constitutional cough."[90] In their first conversation, the young Edward swears to John that he will protect Mary from these fortune hunters. As the luck of sensation novels would have it, John does receive his financial legacy and does indeed die young by virtue of his constitutional tubercular one. Edward Arundel keeps his boyhood promise to John to protect his daughter—by marrying her. However, after Edward receives a head injury during their honeymoon, John's worst fears are realized: Mary is left at the mercy of her conniving relatives, who refuse to believe that she is legitimately married to Arundel because of his absence (he has been injured while away from Mary and out of his senses for a large portion of the novel). Latching onto the excuse of her disgrace as a fallen woman, they lock her away in a shack for two years in order to capitalize on her inheritance by planting seeds of a rumor that she has killed herself in despair over her abandonment.

Although it is her scheming uncle, Paul Marchmont, who develops this plan, he is only capable of enacting it through the assistance of Olivia Arundel née Marchmont. Olivia embodies all *East Lynne*'s rivalries rolled into one, for she has always been passionately in love with her own cousin and Mary's husband, Edward Arundel, and bitterly begrudges Mary her marriage. To make matters worse, Mary's father had, before his death, naively married Olivia, not out of love but in the belief that she would serve as a good mother-figure to Mary. Olivia is thus Mary's legal guardian and bitterest enemy, and it is only through her facilitation that Paul can gain access to Mary to do away with her.

When Olivia first meets Mary, the narrator contemplates Olivia's character:

> What was it in Olivia Arundel's handsome face from which those who looked at her so often shrank, repelled and disappointed? . . . Perhaps it was too much like a marble mask, exquisitely chiseled, but wanting in variety of expression. The handsome mouth was rigid; the dark grey eyes had a cold light in them. . . . Heaven help the wretched creature who had appealed from minor tribunals to *her* mercy! Heaven help delinquents of every kind whose last lingering hope had been in her compassion![91]

Although Olivia fulfills what she believes to be her duties to Mary as a step-mother, and rarely ever acts with overt cruelty toward her, the apathy and lack of sympathy she displays is depicted as equally as damaging as Cornelia's outright antipathy in *East Lynne*. For Braddon, this is the very point. Women cannot withstand a world of patriarchal hegemony—writ large in the melo-drama-style villainy of Paul Marchmont—without a *heartfelt* unity toward one another. Animosity of the sort Isabel encounters is not necessarily the only evil facing women in a world where the decks are so highly stacked against them. In an intrinsically misogynistic society, she indicates, women have need of sincere emotional bonds with one another; apathy, she reveals, can be just as deleterious as antipathy. In fact, Braddon's novel seems to invoke the truism "apathy, not hate, is the opposite of love." If powerful female interactions via rivalry structure *East Lynne* (albeit in their negative capacities), *John Marchmont's Legacy* shows that the complete lack of notice or concern of women for other women leaves them with precisely—nothing. As the narrator continues after describing Olivia's character, "Perhaps Mary Marchmont vaguely felt something of all this. At any rate, the enthusiasm with which she had been ready to regard [her] cooled suddenly beneath the winter in that pale, quiet face."[92] Thus, Braddon's work depicts no fiery, impassioned hatred like that found in *East Lynne*, but only the empty stasis of winter, where abeyance and belay are Hell rather than a mere Purgatory (and which Braddon portrays as more insidiously vitiating). Whereas Wood indicts a society that denies female unity by showing the potency of female rivalry, Braddon's social critique succeeds by depicting the deflated potentialities left open even in the absence of such animosity, and this absence is more poignant, perhaps, than even *East Lynne's* melodrama, for the timbre of *John Marchmont's Legacy* is overwhelmingly cold, quiet, and a bit uneventful. The main character, after all, spends most of the novel *out of* its textual bounds, hidden away from even the reader's eye in an isolated hut. Olivia and Mary—both desperately in love with Edward (who ignores the former and seems rather inept at protecting the latter), and both manipulated and controlled by Paul Marchmont—fade into the background, while Paul and Edward become its major actors. Moreover, although Mary and Olivia by all rights ought to recognize the similarity of their circumstances at the hands of variously ignorant and evil men, there is instead simply a void of understanding between them, and both women are ruined because of it. As the narrator reflects:

> It was thus that these two women met: while one was but a child
> in years; while the other was yet in the early bloom of womanhood:

these two, who were predestined to hate each other, and inflict suffering upon each other in the days that were to come. It was thus that they thought of one another; each with an unreasonable dread, an undefined aversion gathering in her breast.[93]

After two years, Arundel discovers Mary's location, after her guilt-ridden stepmother Olivia acknowledges her role in the kidnapping and shows Arundel where she has been. Olivia goes mad by the novel's end, wracked with guilt for her part in the events. Much like Cornelia's hindsight recognition of the difference that friendship could have made in Isabel's life, Edward and Mary are reunited, but Mary soon dies from an unnamed disease that may be understood as the constitutional "legacy" of the novel's title. Descriptions of Mary invoke the rhetoric of consumption early on and tag her as incapable (like Isabel) of withstanding such an isolating environment. Mary is described early in the novel as having, even from childhood, a "morbidly sensitive, rather than strong" character, that "stored up" "dim poetic sentiments."[94] Later in the work, she is described once again as "morbidly sensitive," and then her empathetic potency is explained in language almost identical to that used to describe Isabel's personality: "She had a subtle and intuitive comprehension of other people's feelings, derived from the extreme susceptibility of her own."[95] Like many consumptives, she is unable to bear up under average worldly concerns. In response to Olivia's dutiful educational instruction, she

seemed to get weaker and paler; and her heavy head drooped wearily under the load of knowledge which it had been made to carry, like some poor sickly flower, oppressed by the weight of dew-drops, which would have revivified a hardier blossom.[96]

In addition to creating the empty air of apathy that wafts desultorily through this story in place of the palpable and powerful animosity whose weighty presence pervades *East Lynne*, Braddon takes her tale and its protagonist to the upper extremities of isolation, as Mary is horrifyingly shut away from all human contact for two years. Braddon uses this complete isolation from interpersonal interactions to indict a social system that does not encourage women's sincere support of one another. In fact, Edward's incompetence in locating Mary suggests that heteronormative relationships are essentially *incapable* of offering the sort of spiritual connection women need to traverse life successfully.[97] In stark juxtaposition to the early-century bubble of safety provided by Helen's consumptive status and concomitant separation from the "scourge" of Lowood, Mary's isolation (like Isabel's before her) in fact stokes the flames of her tubercular legacy and causes her death. Both Brontë and Braddon (along with Wood) subtly insist upon the redemptive potential of homosocial bonds into narratives apparently offering tales of heteronormative propriety. Bequeathed a constitution unable to withstand such dismay and isolation, Mary dies, another sensational sacrifice on the altar of hegemony—an altar that both Wood and Braddon subtly destabilize with risk encounters even as their narratives purportedly parade sexual chastity and marital fidelity.

"A Terrible Tension in the Air": Female Bonds in *The Story of a Modern Woman*

A similarly overt awareness of a systemic evil that prevents women from recognizing their shared oppression pervades Ella Hepworth Dixon's *The Story of a Modern Woman*. In Dixon's novel, class is an ineffectual barrier to invisible microbes, which link the women in the novel through contagion, rendering their shared interests starkly visible. Much as Brontë, Braddon, and Wood deftly mold tubercular tropes to serve their messages about women, rather than simply mirroring scientific discourse, Dixon, while living just in the wake of germ theory's popular cultural hold, selects this rhetoric from a *multiplicity* of options in order to make her case. Dixon's novel, published in 1894, came well after germ theory was widely accepted in the 1870s and '80s and nearly fifteen years after Robert Koch discovered the precise microbe that caused tuberculosis. However, as mentioned earlier, consumption's perplexing mode of transmission caused it to remain something of an etiological mystery, and while many late-century articles espoused the contagiousness of the disease, almost as many continued to insist upon an (often simultaneous) inherited, predisposed weakness to the microbe, an argument that often culminated in eugenicist discourse.[98] As late as 1912, famed Victorian statistician Karl Pearson devoted an entire book, *Tuberculosis, Heredity, and the Environment*, to the topic. After a great deal of statistical analysis, he concludes the text by explaining that eugenicists like himself have "something better to propose" than mere etiological considerations.[99] He continues:

No one can study the pedigrees of pathological states, insanity, mental defect, albinism &c., collected by our Laboratory, without being struck by the large proportion of tuberculous members—occasionally the tuberculous man is a brilliant member of our race—but the bulk of the tuberculous belongs to stocks which we want *ab initio* to discourage. Everything which tends to check the multiplication of the unfit, to emphasize the fertility of the physically and mentally healthy, will *pro tanto* aid Nature's method of reducing the [tuberculosis] death rate. That is what the Eugenist proclaims as the "better thing to do," and £1,500,000 spent in encouraging healthy [bloodlines] would do more than the establishment of a sanatorium in every township.[100]

Even into the twentieth century, then, the mythos of tuberculosis pervaded social discourse, hovering miasmatically and persistently in spite of the bacteriological rhetoric that was taking center stage in regard to most diseases. While no one could deny that tuberculosis was associated with a bacterium, its mysterious epidemiological pathway kept the notion of a hereditary weakness—often construed in this late period as an inherited susceptibility *to* the bacillus—alive. "This impaired power of resistance," one 1897 article proclaims, "may be the result of heredity."[101] The author, like Pearson, concludes that it is "unfortunate that such matters are so little considered in marrying. . . . It is not that the disease is inherited, but the vulnerable tissues, the feeble resistive powers, render the offspring an easy prey to the ubiquitous bacillus."[102] In spite of the continuing viability of the rhetoric of "inherited constitutional weakness" that built upon earlier romantic tropes of consumption, Dixon insists on a *purely* microbial narrative that does not align perfectly with contemporaneous or even contemporary scientific understandings. In fact, even today, most cases of tuberculosis involve some element of immunosuppression along with bacterial contamination; thus, *The Story of a Modern Woman* cannot be read as simply allying itself to some contemporary or natural scientific "fact." Rather, Dixon pointedly selects the socioscientific elements that suit her purpose of revealing the inextricable union of all women in society, whether they recognize this connection or not. Thus, just in the era where one might expect a heightened sense of the value of Helen Burns's quarantined bubble of a morally and microbially pure space for women, Dixon instead insists upon delineating interpersonal female connections *from within* the messy, microbial world of tuberculosis.

Near the end of the novel, the aristocratic Alison Ives, the best friend of Mary Earle, dies of what would have been termed "galloping" consumption.[103] Devoted to charity work, Alison visits the hospital at which her fiancé, Dr. Dunlop Strange, works and becomes intrigued by the nameless "Patient Twenty-seven." Unbeknownst to her, Patient Twenty-seven is her fiancé's ex-mistress and is dying of consumption, contracted after she is spurned and throws herself into a river. The trope of a ruined woman throwing herself into a river, as well as the more general notion of fallen women dying, is hardly novel, of course, but Dixon plays out the fallen woman trope microbiologically.[104] Alison learns Patient Twenty-seven's story after spending an afternoon with her in the hospital, and it is from her that Alison acquires her rapid and terminal form of consumption. She then dies a violent and feverish death, horrified to the end by the knowledge she has gained of her fiancé's cruelty to another woman—which, the novel makes clear, is essentially cruelty to all women, as an oppressed group.

In *Jane Eyre*, Helen Burns's consumption serves to mark her as "classed" above her peers; in *East Lynne*, Isabel Vane's sole friend is her lower-class servant Joyce, the only female character who does not threaten the middle-class order of marriage and heterosexual relationships controlled by patriarchal authority. Alison Ives's contact with a lower-class woman, by contrast, leads to her death, as Patient Twenty-seven is infected with a disease that knows no cultural bounds. No longer, it seems, can women find safety in class barriers.[105] Indeed, Alison's contamination teaches her that "male sexual involvement with the lower-classes cannot be separated from marital sexuality."[106] Isabel's death is the result of her degenerate extramarital sex, but it is also the result of a cultural ideology that isolates women from one another and fails to value their homosocial bonds. Alison's death, by contrast, results most immediately from innocent physical contact with a woman who has contagious mycobacteria in her lungs but in fact stems from the transgressions of her own fiancé, whose heartless treatment of women results in Patient Twenty-seven's contraction of tuberculosis. Thus, whereas Isabel and Mary die due to a constitutional inability to withstand the isolation enforced upon them by a society that cannot endure the erosion of male authority, Alison dies through her very unity with other women who are similarly vulnerable to the dangers of the abuse of masculine authority. Rather than finding companions in those who are far enough below her social class so as to render them less threatening to the hegemonic patriarchal order, as Isabel does, or finding an idealistic space *outside* of class, as Helen and Jane do, Alison finds herself involuntarily united to women of all classes through the uniform feminine condition of vulnerability to men who treat them as nothing but commodities necessary for their own growth and proliferation. Ironically, the female camaraderie Isabel desperately seeks in *East Lynne* is found in *The Story of a Modern Woman* in women's vulnerability to the very hegemonic patriarchal authority that ultimately kills Isabel.

In her novel, Dixon constructs a brutal dystopia that tethers itself to microbial discourse in ways that contradict the earlier discourses of tuberculosis. There *is* no space outside of class, Dixon's text insists, and there is no point in representing female death at the hands of men as a form of beautiful martyrdom. Thus, whereas Isabel Vane (and Helen Burns and Mary Marchmont) dies the fictive "good" death from consumption, Alison dies a more realistically terrible, painful death, complete with the most feared aspects of delirium, pain, and expulsion of bodily fluids. When Mary first leaves the Alison's sickroom, all she can contemplate are Alison's "blisters" and the "emetics" she will need "if [Alison's] . . . bronchial tubes fill . . . up."[107] Later, the "clammy perspiration" on Alison's brow leaves her hair "damp" and clumped on her forehead.[108] Shortly before Alison's death, Mary notes that "the choking mucus" in Alison's chest is beginning to suffocate her.[109] Alison also comments on the edema that has developed in her hands and feet. She shows one foot to Mary as an example, and Mary agrees internally that it is "quite disfigured."[110] While such descriptions are hardly grotesque by contemporary standards, textual contemplation of an aristocratic woman's failing organs would have been surprising by nineteenth-century standards, especially considering the popular image of the peaceful, wasting consumptive death that elided embodied realities of the illness. But however lost such grotesqueness may be on the modern sensibility, it illustrates a marked divergence from the standard romantic consumptive death. Rather than a peaceful wasting away, Alison's death is bloated with the weight and omnipresence of contagion—bloated, that is, with the palpable effects and weight of male transgression and misuse of women. The profusion of visible signs of disease importantly indicates the grossly pervasive injustice of masculine authority over women, which paradoxically links all women together as equal victims of oppression, for which solidarity of sex is the only possible solution. Even from her own deathbed, Alison does not view Patient Twenty-Seven as a rival, in spite of their connection through Dr. Strange. Instead, she pities her as a fellow sufferer:

> It can't be nice to die in a hospital, can it? The ugly, long ward, those ghastly twitching faces on the pillows, the students star-

ing at you. . . . He made her what she was . . . that wretched creature was a respectable girl . . . when she first saw him. No, it isn't a pretty world.[111]

Ultimately, in *The Story of a Modern Woman,* consumptive death has nothing to do with female purity or lack thereof and everything to do with *male* transgression. Rather than creating a safe space for female homosociality through the pure moral vessel of tuberculosis as Brontë does, or repurpose tubercular rhetoric to indict female isolation in a patriarchal society, as Wood and Braddon do, Dixon changes the conversation entirely. Whereas Isabel and Mary Marchmont die due to a constitutional inability to withstand the isolation enforced upon them by a society that cannot endure preclusion of male authority, Alison dies through her very unity with other women who are similarly vulnerable to the dangers of the abuse of masculine authority. Alison finds herself—as Wood and Braddon represent their characters to have been all along—involuntarily united to women through the uniform condition of female vulnerability to male authority. By selecting a disease narrative that emphasizes bare microbial pathways and disregards subjective weaknesses or individual differences, Dixon poignantly gestures toward the necessary and unavoidable solidarity of sex. Thus, the female camaraderie desperately sought by Isabel and sorely missed by Mary Marchmont is recovered and resuscitated in *The Story of a Modern Woman* in the depiction of all women's vulnerability to the oppressive gender norms that ultimately kill Isabel and Mary.

East Lynne is preoccupied with the threat of female transgression of patriarchal hegemony and treats Isabel's death as warranted, in accordance with its readers' ideology. Yet it nevertheless incriminates the social system that catalyzes her death; while women are punished for threatening the status quo, they are posited to have done so because of the intolerability of the system, which demands their absolute isolation from one another. *The Story of a Modern Woman* approaches the same issue of women's oppression by men from a different angle, as women are in community *by virtue of* their mistreatment at the hands of men. Consumption represents male transgressions that permeate class boundaries and unite women who are uniformly threatened by the patriarchy. Working within the social and scientific milieu of their day, then, both texts critique patriarchal authority, opening space for discourse in which female camaraderie is the weapon of choice against male authority.

In Hepworth Dixon's text, "feminine unsightliness and imminent death are . . . imaged as the physical signs of male pleasure-seeking."[112]

The recognition of male oppression and misuse of women figure heavily in the scientifically influenced understanding of contagion. Athena Vrettos has pointed out the significant "power of illness to . . . transgress somatic and psychic boundaries . . . to link disparate groups of people through the process of contagion."[113] The profusion of visible signs of disease indicates the grossly pervasive injustice of male authority over women, which links all women together through their victimization.

Indeed, it is Alison's contamination that prompts Alison and Mary to recognize their unity. "Promise me," Alison begs of Mary, "that you will never, never do anything to hurt another woman."[114] In her fatal illness, Alison has realized that, however involuntary her unity with other women is, it issues from a shared vulnerability to men; if women educate one another about this threat and support each other in community and camaraderie, so much the better for the entire sex. Mary responds affirmatively, claiming that the time for a community of women "is dawning. . . . All we modern women are going to help each other, not to hinder."[115] The very air, the narrator chimes in, held "a terrible tension," and seems "charged with feminine emotion" as they make this pact.[116] Thus, rather than the individual vector of degeneracy that Isabel's consumption represents in her transgressive sexual acts, Alison's consumption is represented as a communal consequence of male authority and as a revolting illustration of its deleterious effects on women. Yet it is the very deleterious effects of male authority that unite women, drawing them out of the externally imposed state of isolation that Isabel's and Mary's consumptive deaths subversively critique. *The Story of a Modern Woman* appropriates the metaphors of consumption used in *East Lynne* and *John Marchmont's Legacy*—using new scientific understandings of the disease—to insist on the fact that women are vitally connected to one another by the very system that insists they be tied to men—men who inevitably abuse and exaggerate the necessity of their authority over women. Importantly, Dixon's selection of simple microbial etiologies and her disregard for the discourse of inherited weakness precludes a reductive ending to the novel. *The Story of a Modern Woman* does not end happily, but rather uncertainly, with Mary Earle standing on a hill, staring into the horizon, and contemplating the potential of female life at the *fin-de-siècle*. In some ways, then, Dixon's novel comes full circle, resting at a place of reflective consideration on the cusp of a new era, as Bronte's does. Dixon's insistence on purely microbial pathways seems to purposefully sidestep the easy answers afforded by eugenicist arguments such as Karl Pearson's. For Dixon, the answer for women in the dawn of a new era cannot be so simplistic as to suggest that bloodlines be cleaned up. Rather, her microbial narrative illuminates pathways of connectivity but does not suggest simplistic means of resolution. Ultimately, Dixon indicates (as Mary repeats Tennyson's words over and over in the novel's final pages), we must simply continue on, "to strive, to seek, to find, and not to yield."[117] In this late-century novel, then, the beauty and power of female camaraderie is resurrected from its stasis, but revealed in all its complexity, and Mary is able to reassure Alison in her dying moments that "our time is dawning. . . . All we modern women are going to help each other, not to hinder. And there is a great deal to do!"[118]

4

Tainted Love

Venereal Disease, Morality, and the Contagious Disease Acts in Ibsen's *Ghosts* and Hardy's *The Woodlanders* and *Jude the Obscure*

It would be curious to [learn] . . . how much of the sickening essence . . . Mr. Hardy has thought his . . . public could stomach.

—Margaret Oliphant, *Blackwood's*, 1896

Ghosts is a medical clinic for the treatment of diseases arranged for the stage by Henrik Ibsen, the eminent authority on human nature.

—*New York Evening World*, January 29, 1903

Like all of Mr. Hardy's work, *The Woodlanders* contains much that is positively repulsive. . . . and yet we read him because of something that lays hold of the imagination lightly but firmly.

—*The Critic*, April 16, 1887

We know [Ibsen's] defects, his lack of humor, of charm, his *bourgeois* imagination . . . his lack of style; and we also know his power, relentless grasp of realities, his cruelty kin to that of the surgeon who heals as he pains.

—*The Sun*, January 27, 1903

The Horror!

A repulsive attraction, a fixation with the lurid, exposed underbelly of "decent" society: throughout the nineteenth century, critics repeatedly described both Thomas Hardy and Henrik Ibsen in this manner. Victorian critical assessments of these authors in many ways parallel the love-to-hate assessments of reality TV shows made by contemporary media critics and popular audiences. While opponents and supporters of both men scrawled their aversion with one queasy hand, they illustrated a surprising ambidexterity as the other hand almost universally lauded the authors as geniuses and masters of the craft. Even Margaret Oliphant, so famously horrified by Hardy's "impious" and "foul" books that dwell in "dark corners where the amateurs of filth find garbage to their taste," made sure to qualify her critique in asserting that the true horror of the displays stemmed from their origination in a "Master's hand."[1]

Janus-faced estimations of Hardy and Ibsen persist even today. I personally can vividly recall being confronted at a party by a man—an academic, no less—who demanded an explanation for my interest in Hardy, who was, in his estimation, the single most depressing author in existence. Norwegians have expressed similar sentiments about Ibsen, even as they tout him as a national icon. Strangely, when asked to defend my enjoyment of Hardy and Ibsen, I often find myself at a loss for words; but there is something in the work of both men that demands witness, even as it repulses. Their texts arrest the reader in a responsive limbo, compelling and yet repelling in their alluring degradation and scenes of degraded allure. Something about Jude's story attracts—haunts, even—and readers have continued to follow his morose footsteps even unto the threshold of the closet where his children hang. Likewise, there is something in Hedda Gabler's manic search for meaning—her desperate desire to slough off the skin of her own ennui even if it means blowing her brains out—that strikes true to us, rather stymied in the middle echelons of class as the majority of us are. Somehow, a bullet to the head isn't enough to kill our empathy with Hedda's dilemma, and in these moments we find the source of the authors' success.

By tapping into the hauntingly tragic, the dangerously dirty, and the (hitherto) unspeakably depraved, Ibsen and Hardy have held audiences in attentive stasis for more than a century and a half. There is active resistance—aversion, even—to their entrancing worlds, but this resistance also *engages* with dark truths that might otherwise be ignored. As William Archer said of Ibsen's *A Doll's House*, "Many—perhaps the majority—violently resented the novel experience, but they could not elude it."[2] Through the dirty, the strange, and the diseased, Hardy and Ibsen recycled dingy and dismal realities to force reader attention to the marginalized and disenfranchised groups that undergird and bolster "polite society." What is there in the artistry of both authors that requires abiding the gutters behind the prim manor houses? Why do both men insist that, as Hardy put it, "if a way to the better there be, it exacts a full look at the worst"?[3] What is it about the foul and the filthy that gives their work cultural heft—such heft that even those who deplored their indecency themselves harnessed the rhetorical power of pathological and sanitary discourse?

Curiously, Hardy and Ibsen have virtually never been critically compared, except in passing, in spite of significant parallels between them.[4] For one thing, both men lived during roughly the same time period (Ibsen, 1828–1906; Hardy, 1840–1928) and were thus exposed to similar cultural concerns; while Ibsen's Norway was arguably somewhat disconnected from the cultural milieu of Victorian Britain, Ibsen spent most of his productive years in Germany and Italy and thus shared a much closer cultural context with Hardy than might otherwise have been the case.[5] In addition, although the men seem never to have met or corresponded, they shared a common literary circle, as both were in close correspondence with Edmund Gosse and William Archer.[6] Most importantly, both men took up many of the same thematic concerns: questions of social mobility, the role of women in a changing society, and—my focus in this paper—the righteousness of extant systems of social propriety. Finally, both men were keenly attuned to the scientific discourse of their day and often used it to work to serve their own ends and subvert systems of social propriety.

I intend this chapter to serve in part as a first foray into the uncharted territory connecting Hardy's and Ibsen's work. I focus, however, on the underbelly of their work—the sticky, messy, tangled-up subject matter that both used as vessels for their thematic aims. In addressing two of the most famous and controversial authors of the late-Victorian era, I establish in this chapter the factors underlying their choices to use disease—here, sexually transmitted disease—as a powerful channel to probe and critique broader social conditions. In the previous chapters, I have shown texts and authors that posited isolation not as safe and pure, but as stifling, and possibly disease-ridden itself. In Defoe and Shelley, readers are privy to the futility of quarantine, and, particularly through Defoe, its potential to allow for greater disease growth through stagnant festering. James inverts this dynamic in his depiction of a young woman who chooses isolation *from* this risk-averse society in order to counter its very insistence on purity through avoidance of risk encounters. The female authors in the last chapter deftly use disease to show that isolation itself is the disease society ought to be most concerned with. This thematic trajectory leads nicely to Ibsen's and Hardy's use of disease, as both authors weave these strands of isolation, risk aversion, and questions of social progress together in their considerations of the performance of moral purity in a socially rigid age—considerations that, as I will show, are communicated through the vehicle of the diseases coded as most socially *im*pure, venereal disease. My analyses reveal in Ibsen's case the spiritual anemia of social and moral isolation, and in Hardy's the salvific potential of engagement in the social world, even if it means crossing moral and pathogenic boundaries.

Indeed, both Hardy and Ibsen could be characterized as "lovable literary renegades," insofar as their work remained popular even as it consistently challenged the status quo—both by featuring incendiary subject matter and by raising the question of what could be printed or even discussed in "proper" social discourse—and thus incurred critical ire. That Hardy abandoned novel writing in reaction to critical assessments of *Jude the Obscure* is a famous (if dubious) literary event. Arguably less famous, anecdotally at least, are the reactions to Ibsen's equally contentious works—works that often dealt with many of the same themes as Hardy's novels.[7]

Like many of Hardy's texts, the 1891 English debut of *Ghosts*, the third of Ibsen's so-called problem-plays, was met with critical outrage.[8] George Bernard Shaw collected many of the negative reviews in his *Quintessence of Ibsenism*: "absolutely loathsome and fetid," "gross, almost putrid," "literary carrion," and "naked loathsomeness" were some of the milder epithets attached to the production.[9] Timothy Carlo Matos describes the backlash against the play and its playwright as "one of the most inflammatory theatrical quarrels in European theatre history," resulting in approximately five hundred printed reviews and reactions.[10] One oft-cited review, which appeared in *Daily Telegraph*, deemed the play an "open drain . . . a loathsome sore unbandaged . . . a dirty act done publicly; a lazar house with all its doors and windows open."[11] The characters that populate the play, the reviewer continued, "expectorate . . . in public, and air on the stage matters that a blind beggar would hide under his patches."[12] Notably, Matos devotes an entire article to exploring the curious fact that reviewers often responded to *Ghosts* with vitriolic attacks using language typically associated with contagious diseases, while virtually none used such language in assessing *Enemy of the People* (first produced in 1893), a play whose action centers around a cholera outbreak. Matos's ultimate assertion is that cholera, though contagious, does not threaten the public's sense of decency in the same way as an overt discussion of syphilis, the disease of interest in *Ghosts*.

Matos's point is well taken. Depictions of sexual impropriety and sexually transmitted diseases ("STDs") obviously contravened Victorian social decorum. In fact, Evert Sprinchorn notes that the very word *syphilis* did not appear in print until 1901.[13] However, I would expand upon Matos's working hypothesis and argue further that critics analyzed Hardy and Ibsen in language that made broad use of epidemiological discourse, whether discussing a range of their texts or the authors' fictional creations and thematic interests as a whole. Of specific interest here is my claim that critical discourse took this approach because of the significant cultural significance of disease and infection in the bacteriological age, collateral that Hardy and Ibsen strategically cashed in on to bolster their socially subversive claims. Disease in their works points unwaveringly at a *diseased moral society*, not mere agentless microbes, as the true etiological source. In doing so, their works also make claims about societal admonitions regarding moral and bacterial purity, turning their arguments back upon themselves to show that, paradoxically, these admonitions actually degrade society through their misguided aims. Hardy went even farther, specifically upholding diseased and contaminated relationships as more natural and potentially fruitful than anything as unnatural and impossible as a perfectly sterile union.

The authors' appropriation of disease discourse is so complex in its rhetorical and thematic maneuvers—folding over and over itself like so many polypeptides within a protein—that contemporary critics decrying the foul filth of "Ibsenism" and Hardyism often found themselves trapped within—and reliant on—their discursive web. Hardy and Ibsen so deftly repurposed disease that their own thematic claims became culturally contagious, even in the mouths of naysayers. Indeed, whatever power Hardy and Ibsen found in discourses of pathology, reviewers evidently found equally persuasive, as they made similar linguistic choices in analyzing their work. For example, one essay, aptly titled "The Ibsen Bacillus," insists that "the pity of" Ibsen's popularity "is that a man who might have done much better should have started or re-started a bacillus, which has infected . . . his pretentious admirers."[14] Another reviewer likened *Ghosts* to spoiled food: a "highly Rancid drama" for the author of "More Morbid than Ibsen."[15] Of Hardy, one reviewer claimed that his work was full of "nauseous cant . . . false sentiment . . . vulgar ostentation . . . probably . . . due to evil influence."[16]

Reviewers also often spoke critically of Hardy using broadly scientific and medical, rather than specifically pathological, discourse. Perhaps, to take Matos's point, this is because Hardy less overtly cast infectious disease as a central structuring device for his novels. However, the use of scientific terminology in contemporary reviews of Hardy's work speaks to the undercurrent of scientific and medical discourse that helps unify his novels. For one reviewer, *Far From the Madding Crowd* was "a mutilated" pastoral.[17] Another deplored his "dissection" of the protagonists in *Return of the Native*.[18] In *Jude the Obscure*, "the anatomy of suffering" Hardy laid out "becomes vivisection," a term that evokes the issue of medical dissection of animals that was actively being debated late in the century.[19] One reviewer in particular warned against "contamin[ating]" young girls' minds with *Jude the Obscure*.[20] As this chapter will show, contamination was readily associated in the Victorian era with sexually transmitted disease, and one of Hardy's earliest reviewers lamented that "the author's powers" were not "extended, instead of being prostituted to the purpose of idle prying into the ways of wickedness."[21]

If Hardy and Ibsen were veritable "bacilli" due to their contagious influences, there is no doubt that they infected the very reviewers who critiqued them using similar disease rhetoric. Ultimately, I argue that Hardy's and Ibsen's treatment of the contagious nature of the illnesses in their texts reveals the complex nature of their social critiques, as both authors repurpose medical and scientific viewpoints to make their case. Indeed, a careful reading of Ibsen's *Ghosts* (1881) and Hardy's *The Woodlanders* (1887) shows that in the post-germ-theory world and the dawning era of bacteriology both authors injected disease into that most intimate of human relationships—marriage and sexual partnerships—precisely to *invert* disease discourse. Rather than depicting scrupulous cleanliness, whether of mind or body, as a laudable goal, both sought to show purity as confoundingly self-contaminating. *Ghosts* and *The Woodlanders* illustrate vividly that those who try the hardest to uphold socially approved standards of propriety in fact contaminate society with an infectious and insidious moral degeneracy.

Risky Business: The Contagious Disease Acts in Context

Both *Ghosts* and *The Woodlanders* appeared at a time when social constructs surrounding sexually transmitted disease were changing. In Britain, a series of legal sanctions called The Contagious Disease Acts were enacted in 1864 in an attempt to control the spread of syphilis. Any woman suspected of being a prostitute could be forcibly detained by police and undergo "compulsory instrumental introspection of her person" in search of signs of syphilis, which, if found, allowed police to incarcerate the woman in a hospital for up to three months.[22] The process entitled women to "no jury, no counsel" and no ability to ask the apprehending officer "what . . . his 'good cause' " was.[23] Importantly, the Contagious Disease Acts ("CDA") were based on similar, earlier legislation in France and Sweden—syphilis "was rampant in Scandinavia in the 1880s."[24] The Contagious Disease Acts—which situated prostitutes as the sole vectors of venereal diseases, with syphilis being the chief concern—were repealed in 1886. The change came out of a growing awareness that, without men to traffic in prostitutes, venereal disease could not spread—an awareness I argue is necessarily linked to the predictable epidemiological pathways made apparent by germ theory.[25] Although *Ghosts* was written five years before the repeal of the Acts, resistance and repeal efforts had been underway almost since their inception. Before the repeal efforts succeeded, however, the CDA was founded on and perpetuated a worldview in which "prostitutes were seen as both physically and morally responsible for the spread of venereal disease. They were seen not merely as agents of transmission but as inherently diseased, if not the disease itself."[26] Indeed, even as Ibsen and Hardy used syphilis as a vehicle for their concerns about the ideological moral purity of the hearth and home, those in the Pro-CDA camp also conflated prostitution itself with disease: "It is a necessary evil only in the same sense that poverty and disease are necessary evils, and it is almost as impossible to eradicate one as the others."[27]

The subject was incendiary. Entire periodicals were devoted to the topic of repeal, *The Shield* being the most famous. Indeed, since their passage, the CDA were instantly a topic of hugely publicized debates in print, usually hinging on assertion or disavowal of the same set of topics (e.g., that the Acts did or did not implicitly isolate women alone as transmitters of the disease; whether or not men ought, by rights, also to be policed; whether or not the Acts allowed for abuses of power when it came to police inspection of women's bodies) rather than disputes over the veracity or interpretation of certain facts. Somewhat akin to vaccination debates today, both sides of the CDA debates focused on the same sets of concerns, with each party's arguments essentially amounting to claims of "no they don't" or "yes they do." The result in periodicals is therefore dizzyingly repetitive; yet this insistent repetition of the same ideas renders in great clarity the precise issues that concerned Victorians about the Acts. The table of contents of one such treatise summarizes the issues volleyed back and forth quite well:

I. Should we treat enthetic diseases at all?

II. Ought they to be treated by the Government at the public expense?

III. Contagious Disease Acts

(a) Sanitary results[28]

(b) Moral and social effects[29]

(c) Do [the laws] increase clandestine prostitution?

(d) Do they interfere unduly with the liberty of the subject?

(e) Are they a form of license of prostitution?

(f) Is their inequality as applying to only one sex a valid objection?[30]

Given the biopolitical scope of this book, as well as the aims of the literature discussed here, I will focus briefly on the portions of the debate that dealt with moral and social justifications and outcomes (points I, II, III[b] and III[d–f]), rather than the aspects of the debates that addressed its efficacy or lack thereof (points III[a] and III[c]). To the first two main points, CDA supporters argued that compulsory vaccination, among other public health mandates, set a precedent for such legislation.

In large part, the CDA as a whole were a relic of Victorian gender binaries. Opponents of the Acts were well aware of the double standards the CDA relied upon, and were quick to point them out to the reading public. One pamphlet puts the matter thusly:

Male civilians are not under such despotism; and the Act is quite silent about them. This may not be marvelous, yet it is infamous. No epithet of scorn and hatred can be too strong for this dastardly favouritism of the male sex. Who are the original seducers of women? Men. Who cause disease in women, though you heal them fifty times? Men.[31]

Another publication on the topic says indignantly, "The way to 'stamp out the disease' is to stamp upon the guilty parties, male and female, the mark of public disapprobation. Frown upon the *men*. Let *them* be hunted up, and exposed, and punished."[32] Yet another echoes these sentiments:

It is not unreasonable to suggest that the surveillance which is proposed should be exercised upon the other sex. Let *them* suffer the monthly indignity. Let the probationary course indicated be applied to *them*. Let the police authorities have *their* names on the roll [of registered offenders], and let *them* be furnished with a certificate of health ere they are set at large. Why is legislation to be all on one side? Why are those who by nature are the weaker, the more sensitive, the more helpless, to be subjected to the gross outrage proposed, and the others escape the ordeal?[33]

In the novel-writing world, Sarah Grand would later address this double standard explicitly in *The Heavenly Twins*. However, as her novel addresses these issues in quite a literal way and does so by promoting the necessity of female sexual education, I have here chosen male authors who took up the cause by addressing Victorian ideas of purity and moral superiority (notions that were integral to the CDA); significantly, the authors I cover here use disease itself as an apt stand-in for these social concerns. Typical of the these particular debates, which allowed for the same facts but debated their biopolitical significance, the pro-CDA pamphleteers merely denied the relevance of the double standard, rather than denying that a double standard existed. As Elizabeth Garrett put it, "There would be force in this objection [regarding double standards] if there were any parallel class among men, but in the absence of any such class," such a double standard is the only legislative option.[34] Conversely, one pamphlet, neatly titled *Some Suggestions for Controlling Men as Well as Women*, lays out clear and practical ways in which a parallel class of men could indeed be identified (this author identifies largely the armed forces—which were recognized by both sides as the most "at risk"—as well as any civilian who customs a sex worker). The practical suggestions in this treatise (requiring men who infect women to financially support their treatment; quarantining all naval officers and requiring them to pass medical examination before landing ashore; examination of new recruits prior to their acceptance to the armed forces) stand as sound evidence to the fact that it would in fact be possible to legislate the policing of male bodies as well as women's. Nevertheless, the author grimly acknowledges that "the public will almost always be on the side of *young* men as opposed to *bad women*," and admits that "we are not sanguine enough to imagine that our suggestions . . . will have much effect."[35]

As I have said, in this chapter I will show the ways that Hardy and Ibsen castigate Victorian middle-class morality. Specifically, I will demonstrate that they do so by inserting disease into "pure" homes, thereby revealing Victorian values of propriety and purity to be meaningless and, in fact, diseased. In the Victorian marital home, the wife's status as the quasi-virginal "angel of the house" was a synecdoche for this middle-class morality. Of course, a married woman obviously had sex and bore children, but the traditional Victorian aversion to female sexual enjoyment is probably one of the best-known stereotypes of the period. Indeed, the very "confinement" of visibly pregnant women attests to the premium Victorian society placed on concealing female participation in the sex act. Yet the married man, by virtue of being male, was seen as possessed by an unbridled and insatiable sexuality. For all intents and purposes, then, family patriarchs had to repress sexual urges directed toward their wives (thanks to the angel-in-the-house construct), but were also viewed (and taught to view themselves) as sexually insatiable and therefore given covert license to enlist the services of prostitutes. This strange alchemical mixture, meant to solidify an ideal of golden purity, in fact resulted in a leaden mess in which "good ladies" lacked desire, but were partnered with "good gentlemen" who overflowed with it.

Prostitution is nothing new, of course, but in this context, middle-class morality was virtually dependent upon the traffic of prostitutes for its very survival. As with the other aspects of the CDA debates, both parties seemingly agreed on this fact, with those supporting the Acts naturalizing it and those arguing for repeal pointing the finger back at both the men who trafficked prostitutes and also the moral codes of Victorian hearth-and-home purity that seemingly justified this traffic. Charles Deakin, for instance, opens his treatise on the defensive against this pointing finger, arguing that "when we say that prostitution is a necessary evil, 'we imply' merely that it will 'always exist so long as the animal part of his nature preponderates in man.' "[36] Those who urged for the repeal of the Acts, however, insisted that this very notion of animalistic men was the problem to begin with. This moral code, positing frigid wives and insatiable husbands, insisted that women as a sex were "supposed to be innately pure," while "at the same time thousands of them were needed to be available to service the sexual needs of men."[37]

Deakins upholds the status quo matter-of-factly, claiming that his opponents "in dealing with this question . . . forget the difference in passion of the two sexes," the difference being that "the sexual instinct is much more powerful in men than in women as a rule."[38] He falls back on medical reasoning to support his point, claiming that male ejaculation inevitably occurs in the form of nocturnal emissions if waking desires are unmet. For

Deakin, such claims are proof that men cannot control their sexual desires, thus rendering prostitution the "necessary evil" he deems it at the beginning of his argument. For their part, those urging the repeal of the Acts sneered in disgust at this theoretical framing, particularly the idea that "a young man is bound, in duty to his body, to consort with harlots"—and, regarding nocturnal emissions, they argue that they promote and enable "chastity" rather than stand as evidence of "a dangerous disease" and indicator of a need for sexual intercourse.[39] Opponents argued that belief in men's uncontrollable urges made possible the CDA, which only served to preserve and enable male vice and make such vice less of a risk encounter via policing women's bodies. The thematic connections to the previous chapters here should be obvious. To enforce the Acts, one tract claims, is only to "fetter [and] degrade" the women it affected, offering them up as veritable sacrifices to the "animal gratification" of men, constituting nothing short of "a gross *pandering* to the worst passions of depraved men."[40] *The Remedy Worse than the Disease* adds to this argument, urging that "forced medical intervention" serves only "to . . . continuance of *the sin* without its penalties [for men], and to an extension of facilities for the perpetration with impunity, of the grossest, vilest vice that heaven can behold."[41] Another tract, boldly titled *The Cure of the Great Social Evil with Special Reference to Recent Laws Delusively Called Contagious Diseases' Acts*, brilliantly elucidates the issue:

> "We must by any severity stop this contagion. You cannot stop it by the ordinary process of law. This sharp malady needs sharp remedies." So far, we might agree. One might expect them to add: "Therefore, we must spy out these respectable family-men, arrest them, cleanse them, and break up the brothels." But instead of this, they reason: "Therefore, by operating on the *women,* whether they like it or no, we must bring about that respectable husbands shall find none but sound harlots in the brothels." For my part, I find this to be a very masculine argument.[42]

The pamphlet *Licencing Prostitution* goes so far as to deem the registration and surveillance of prostitutes nothing short of "enrolling these soul-possessing but hapless victims as slaves."[43] The rancor of the author's inclusion of "soul-possessing" as a relevant qualifier for "victims" is an indicator of the outrage the anti-CDA protestors felt in regard to the Acts. The use of the term *slaves* in the period just after the American Civil War is another. Indeed, many of the treatises note that, in spite of their natural delicacy, "ladies young and old are filled with horror at the outrages offered to their sex, and lay aside reticence" to speak out in protest of the legislation.[44]

As important as the sexual double standard, however, is the fact that the CDA were based on notions of insuperable class boundaries. It was, of course, comforting to believe that sexual vice—in this case venereal disease—could be safely confined to the lower classes and that the sanctity of the middle-class home could be protected simply by regulating the activities of the poor. Writers readily took up the cause of gender and paired it with the obvious issues of class at play in the CDA. Such arguments built upon concerns of gender-based exploitation, claiming that the Acts "encourage vice by making it safe and easy to one *class,* while subjecting another to a cruel and demoralizing espionage."[45] However, as efforts to repeal the Acts came to fruition in the mid-1880s—precisely the period when the field of bacteriology was developing and bolstering understanding of germ theory—parts of the public began to understand that venereal disease spread in part by prostitutes was merely a symptom of a larger and more systemic problem: an ethically diseased society whose standard of morality kept both men and women in a state of sexual repression. In fact, this very belief system also depended upon the idea that the middle class was impervious to the effects of sexual vice, which they imagined to be situated in the lower classes. Many opponents cast the Acts as effectually creating and maintaining a separate class of women solely for male sexual use, and spoke explicitly about this in moving terms. Even those in support of the Acts had difficulties avoiding this implicit creation of an entirely discrete class of women in their very attempts to assuage fears that "ordinary" women could be violated. Over and over, pro-CDA treatises go to great lengths to insist that only "the *common* prostitute is the person we wish to control," and such texts establish elaborate guidelines that aim to systematically identify "who can be fairly included in the term 'common prostitute.' "[46] Numerous pro-CDA tracts reaffirm this language of demarcating the "common prostitute" from other women in support of their claims, assuring readers that "until we are positive that the woman is a prostitute from one or more proofs," she is not medically violated.[47] Indeed, the very act of setting apart this class of women as separate, economically and morally, from others, allowed for sex workers' dehumanizing figuration in pro-CDA discourse.

Those arguing against the Acts particularly highlighted this ideological creation of a class that was somehow separate from the morality, rights, and humanity of other Victorians. They called attention to this specific shift over time—"never before" had even this group of women been set aside as a class that had "lost rights over her own person." Rather, "to violate [sex workers]" in the past "was as criminal as to violate a chaste woman."[48] Other treatises attempted to highlight the classed double standard of the laws, asking, "Which of the advocates of the Act would face such a risk himself, or permit any female relative to be examined with the same speculum used for diseased prostitutes?" in this manner.[49] This last qualification hearkens not only to the penetration-based violation, but also the concern that women could be diseased by the very act of the examination in an era where disinfectant methods were nascent—and especially when their use impacted an obviously vulnerable and exploited population whose personal liberties were already being actively disregarded (recall chapter 3). Evidence of the dehumanizing view of the female sex worker necessary to sustain support of the Acts is indicated by the nature of supporters' rebuttals to these arguments. "Can we be expected to believe," asks one author, "that women whose bodies are free to all the world, will, if examined by a surgeon, feel misery?"[50] When opponents of the Acts raised questions about potential abuses of power on the part of police and doctors, this same class bias was integral to pro-CDA defenses. "It should be remembered," one author expounds, "that the Act is not enforced by common constables, but by superintendents of police, men of tried character, of long standing in the force, almost invariably of middle age, and married," as if these aspects of gender, character, age, and domestic propriety were certain enough insurance against their personal vices. In the same breath, these socio-moral class distinctions are upheld because the police "have no power over any but notorious sinners."[51]

The debate over this creation of an underclass of citizens led naturally to discussions of human rights violations and interference with personal liberty. When the argument focused on double standards, those opposed to the Acts argued for the equal human rights of sex workers, whereas those supportive of the Acts struggled to situate these workers as exempt from certain biopolitical rights. But CDA supporters often then shifted the terms of the debate, arguing that, even allowing that sex workers' human rights were on par with those of others, human liberty at large is always subject to the greater good of the government. As mentioned earlier, vaccination laws were often brought to bear upon this subject. One pamphlet argues:

> If my nextdoor [sic] neighbor chooses to have his drains in such a state as to create a poisonous atmosphere, which I breathe at the risk of typhus and diphtheria, he restricts my just freedom to live . . . threatening my life; if he is to be allowed to let his children go unvaccinated, he might as well be allowed to leave strychnine lozenges about in the way of mine.[52]

"What right has a woman," this same author continues, "suffering from syphilis to continue her trade, blasting her own body and that of her fellow sinners with loathsome disease? Have we a right to interfere with her 'liberty' of administering poison?"[53] Generally, such points were bookended by the conclusion that someone's perceived liberty is always subject to restraint when the common good is at stake, an argument unnervingly reminiscent of the haunting statement in *The Handmaid's Tale* that "better never means better for everyone." Of course, both statements necessarily imply that it is generally worse for those most easily exploited by those in power.

A social machine that defines its own value in a manner that necessitates the patronization of prostitutes surely finds it very convenient to locate vice within these quarters, as the CDA did, rather than in the middle-class home. However, burgeoning awareness of predictable epidemiological patterns of venereal disease threatened to topple the house of cards upon which the CDA was built. Emotional pleas for the "delicate and virtuous mother[s]" and their "helpless infants" infected by middle-class husbands ring with pathetic zeal throughout the CDA pamphlets, demonstrating growing awareness that male sexual vice was not, in fact, limited to the lower classes.[54] Thus, the repeal of the CDA and the prior years of resistance caused a great deal of anxiety, as the push for repeal redirected the manicule of vice toward the seat of patriarchal authority: the middle- and upper-class husband. "Think of the poor dear children!" contaminated with congenital syphilis, more than one tract urges.[55] If "malignant virus" could be "introduced into respectable families," the relevance of Victorian middle-class propriety diminishes, and not simply because of sex workers.[56] For one thing, as Mary Spongberg notes, women ceased to be signifiers in this system, as "the purity of the middle-class female stood for nothing" within the new conceptual framework of syphilis.[57] That is, the original rules of the Victorian gender game posited the ever-virginal mother and wife as the sine qua non of the moral middle-class home. But if pure women could contract syphilis from husbands who were now understood to be infecting them because of their traffic in prostitutes, female purity or the lack thereof no longer assured family purity. Syphilis thus not only ate away at the family unit but also insidiously degenerated any faith in the social mores intended to strengthen family units. Within this decaying system of gender norms and moral standards, female purity did little to bolster the morality of the family and society; indeed, the entire system became a satire of propriety and righteousness, confounding its own ends and corroding from the inside out.

Moreover, doctors, part of the patriarchy themselves, were burdened with the question of where infected men fit into the old-order system of domestic virtue.[58] As J. Alfred Fournier—one of the most famous contemporary medical experts on syphilis, and one of the few doctors devoted to protecting women from the effects of male sexual vice—noted, "a man who, before marriage has contracted syphilis, may become dangerous in marriage in three directions;—*firstly* as husband; *secondly* as father; *thirdly*, as head of the social community which he constitutes by his marriage."[59] But even as Fournier championed the health of women, he betrays his own preoccupation with the unraveling tapestry of domestic propriety that threatened to leave the stronghold of the nation in tatters. Other doctors concerned with the same question recommended privileging domestic ideals over women's safety. Jonathan Hutchison, for example, asserted that "where . . . a social institution as vast as marriage is at stake, the surgeon must not push medical scruples too far."[60] For Hutchison, the danger of syphilis was not half as great as the fact that "anxiety about the disease could lead to regulation of marriage, which 'would be disastrous to social progress and would greatly reduce the sum of human happiness.'"[61] As Andrew Smith points out, "Hutchison d[id] not deny that . . . the man . . . [was] largely responsible for the spread of syphilis; he simply propose[d] its concealment" in order to avoid unnecessary turmoil within the family unit.[62] As Hutchison himself stated, "There can be no duty more imperative, in the exercise of our profession, than that of abstaining from needlessly exciting in the minds of our patients suspicions as to conjugal purity."[63]

Amid this changing epidemiological understanding, the significance of female chastity, manly virtue, the institution of marriage, and the entire idealized domestic space in the middle class all fell into question. As Andrew Smith puts it, within this shifting semiotic system, "the spread of the disease seem[ed] to be a consequence of the inability of the male subject to properly commit to some abstract notion of bourgeois family life."[64] Notably, fictional and nonfictional texts on the subject all seem to "nervously raise" the question of "where real value . . . [is] to be found" if "some socially dominant 'norm' becomes pathologized."[65]

Paradoxically, Hardy and Ibsen repurposed this post-germ-theory understanding of epidemiology but jettisoned its potentially deleterious social implications. That is, rather than seeking to maintain purity and segregation from the ostensibly diseased lower classes, both Hardy and Ibsen evinced an astute epidemiological awareness that disease does not obey class boundaries and showed that belief in the sanctity of the middle class and its values in fact diseased society.

"We Are All Ghosts . . . Abysmally Afraid of the Light": The Impotency of Propriety in *Ghosts*

Ibsen's *Ghosts* depicts the last moments in the life of Osvald Alving, a young painter who returns to Norway from the Continent to live with his mother, Helene. In Osvald's absence, Helene (or Mrs. Alving, as she is more often called in the play) has been planning the establishment of a community orphanage dedicated to the memory of her late husband, Captain Alving. As the play opens, Helene discusses the plans for the orphanage with Pastor Manders, the man she has chosen to handle its business affairs. During their discussion, Helene reveals—after years of pretending the contrary—that her ostensibly ideal and pure home was anything but, for her husband was a drunken and licentious man who made her life miserable. This opening conversation also reveals that Helene once attempted to leave her husband—and that she fled to Pastor Manders, whom she loved, but who instructed her to return home and fulfill her duties as a woman and as a wife, "bear[ing] with humility that cross which a higher power had judged proper."[66] Ever since the crucible of her married experience, Helene has resigned herself to maintaining the illusion of her husband's moral scrupulousness, even participating in his "drinking orgies" to ensure that he and his activities were "ke[pt] . . . at home in the evenings."[67] She also sent Osvald away from the family home to the Continent, ostensibly to keep him from the noxious influence of his father. However, her actions are always also geared to maintain the illusion that her family meets a set of externally defined social mores. She mentions, for instance, that she sent Osvald away precisely when he could comprehend that his home was not as perfect as she wanted it to seem; she "couldn't bear" his presence once he was old enough to "notice things and ask questions."[68] She describes her entire life as an "endless battle . . . fought day after day" to keep the truth of her husband and family a secret from the public and to maintain popular belief in the sanctity of her home.[69] Her life has been spent "doing [her] duty, observing the proprieties."[70]

Like her husband's reputation and the Alving home, Helene Alving's reasons for erecting the orphanage are not what they seem; charity is the least of her concerns. Helene has come up with the idea solely to spend her late husband's fortune—a fortune for which, it bears noting, she was pressured to marry him. Helene has "calculated . . . very carefully" the amount that she must funnel into the orphanage to prevent Oswald from "inherit[ing] a single thing from his father" and his life of vice and libertinism.[71] Of course, she adds that it also serves to "kill any rumors, and sweep away any misgivings" as to her husband's status as a pillar of the community.[72]

But Helene's efforts are to no avail, for soon after Oswald returns, he informs her that he has contracted syphilis, and he degenerates mentally by the play's close. Thus, all of Helene's careful attempts to preserve for her son a sense of their family's morally upright status—through avoiding any risky encounters with impropriety—have come to nothing. Likewise, the orphanage, which Manders convinces her not to insure (because "it would be so terribly easy" for the public "to interpret things as meaning that neither [of the two] had a proper faith in Divine Providence"), is destroyed in a fire.[73] Thus, another attempt at propriety literally burns to the ground.

Ibsen's play addresses a very tangible social concern with middle-class morality through the vector of syphilis. Further, and more importantly, it also illustrates the metaphoric significance of syphilis in late Victorian society. As Ross Shideler notes, Ibsen's work often "reflect[s] th[is] tension between . . . public effort[s] to sustain an idealized 'holy family' and the realities of the latter half of the nineteenth century."[74] *Ghosts* makes it clear that Captain Alving's debauchery directly and literally infects his son with his tainted blood—indeed, Osvald says as much when he says that the doctor who diagnosed him stated that "there has been something worm-eaten about [him] since birth."[75] However, it also demonstrates that Helene's attempts to maintain the façade of social propriety within the community are equally complicit in Osvald's decline. This system of supposed morality, built upon overdetermined gender-role performances and illusory class boundaries, ostensibly bolsters the middle class by keeping disease and vice ideologically at bay. But in actuality, its only effect is to inject disease and corruption into the family unit.

Naturally, it would be problematic (as the Victorians were then discovering) to blame middle-class women for the syphilis that their husbands brought home. What *could* Helene have done differently, after all? Of course, since this story presents an alternative ending to *A Doll's House*, one's first instinct is to look to Nora and surmise that Helene could have refused to return to her husband. Notably, such a course of action would unravel the whole play, as Osvald was born after her return, but this only renders

Ibsen's critique that much more scathing. This play and this moral infection of "proper behavior" *shouldn't* exist at all.

To this end, committed to the preservation of her son's belief in his ideal domestic home, Helene repeatedly cries, "What a coward I am!," as she shies away from telling Oswald the truth about his father.[76] Her cowardice persists even when she learns that much of Oswald's despondency results from his belief that he has caused his illness. In spite of his doctor's diagnosis of congenital syphilis, Oswald, deluded by his mother's lies, believes that he must have contracted the disease himself. "If only it had been something inherited . . . something one couldn't have helped," he laments; Helene simply watches him, too fearful even in the face of his utter despair to relieve his suffering with the truth.[77] Only when Oswald prepares to marry Regine (who is his half-sister, conceived as a result of his father's philandering) does Helene finally intervene, for such a union would only breed further disease by spreading the literal contagion of syphilis. She thus shatters the illusion of the happy home as she tells Oswald of his inherited illness, confirming his doctor's original conclusion that "the sins of the fathers are visited upon the children."[78]

Although he is deceived by the "beautiful illusion" of his father's moral purity for much of the play, Oswald is in all respects the clearest-seeing character. When he reflects back on his travels, for example, he bemoans "that glorious, free life out there . . . smeared by *this* filth."[79] The "filth" that besmirches the "glorious, free life" he envisions clearly emanates from the very system of moral propriety that deceived him as to the true nature of his father, a man whose literal filth has noxiously tainted Oswald's own blood. In this light, Oswald's predicted/impending "softening of the brain," a euphemism he embraces as a comforting dilution of a truly ghastly prognosis, seems to be the prognosis for society at large, which willingly deludes itself into a sickly dependence on an outmoded, "worm-eaten" system of ideals.[80] Such ideals seep through bloodlines literally and through families metaphorically, weakening society, turning brains soft through years of unthinking acceptance, and reducing individuals to little more than the invalid Oswald becomes—people who can do nothing for themselves, who are effectively "turned into . . . helpless child[ren] who live at the mercy of society's whims."[81] Indeed, as A. F. Machiraju notes, "the transmission of physical disease from parent to child is a powerful metaphor for the way society transmits its mental diseases of delusion and conformity from one generation to the next."[82] To this end, Machiraju quotes Michael Meyer as claiming that "what *Ghosts* is really about is the devitalizing effect of inherited convention."[83]

Oswald sees all of this for what it is and maintains his glibly morose attitude until his catatonia at the play's conclusion. Helene Alving sees the same things, but only in shades, ghostly transfigurations of the problem that are not ghastly enough to motivate her to action. She explains to Manders her theory that society is built upon nothing more than ghosts:

> I'm inclined to think that we are all ghosts . . . every one of us. It's not just what we inherit from our mothers and fathers that haunts us. It's all kinds of old defunct theories, all sorts of old defunct beliefs, and things like that. It's not that they actually *live* on in us; they are simply lodged there, and we cannot get rid of them. I've only to pick up a newspaper and I seem to see ghosts gliding between the lines. Over the whole country there must be ghosts, as numerous as the sands of the sea. And here we are, all of us, abysmally afraid of the light.[84]

Oswald, however, can see, against the backdrop of the incineration of the orphanage, that "everything will burn" in such a society because, as he sullenly notes, "here am I, burning down too."[85] The effect of propriety on his life is only too present for him. In the face of the imminent annihilation of his intellect, Oswald predicts that his mother, too, will realize the error of her ways soon enough. Just before he slips into dementia, he tells his mother of his desire to die on his own terms, rather than those his father bequeathed to him—he asks that his mother euthanize him rather than allowing him to slip into dementia. He talks about his impending doom and reiterates his request, adding that "meanwhile the sun will be rising. And then you'll know"—a prediction that comes to pass, as in the face of Oswald's catatonic stupor, and against the backdrop of the rising sun, she finally sees the ultimate sterility of her devotion to superficial virtue.[86]

Yet propriety remains first and foremost to Helene up to the bitter end, and the play concludes with a tableau of her indecision in response to her son's dying request. As Osvald slips into a nearly vegetative state, he eerily and without explanation demands, "Mother, give me the sun."[87] The play ends with his repeated demand, "The sun. The sun. . . . The sun. . . . The sun," which haunts Helene as it exposes her continued inability to break free of the ghosts of social mores past. At the play's end, Osvald is trapped in a catatonic stupor, and Helene can only watch as he repeatedly demands that she give him the sun, a task as impossible as success of the system that supposedly knits together "perfect" middle-class families. His final words, "the sun, the sun," set against a sunrise, serve both as a chilling mockery of the system of morality that has birthed every action in the play and as a dark and ghastly prophesy of the fate of future generations—two images in grim, sharp contrast.[88]

Out of the Shadows and into the Light: Inoculative Restitution in *The Woodlanders*

Thomas Hardy's *The Woodlanders* follows the paths of a star-crossed pair: Grace Melbury, an educated, middle-class woman, and Giles Winterbourne, a poor laborer. Like Helene Alving, Grace marries for money and social standing in response to familial pressure. Rather than marrying Giles, her first love, she marries Edred Fitzpiers, a cold and rather ghoulish doctor who collects brains for a hobby. Her parents pressure her to marry Edred "based less on his professional position . . . than on the standing of his family in the county in bygone days."[89] Thus, while Edred is not extremely wealthy, the marriage is still a mercenary one, founded on an attempt to accrue respectability where wealth is wanting and motivated by nothing more than "that touching faith in members of long-established families . . . irrespective of their personal condition or character, which," the narrator notes, "is still found among old-fashioned people in the rural districts," and "had reached its full perfection" in Grace's father.[90]

Like Captain Alving, Edred is chronically unfaithful. Like Helene, Grace tries to leave her husband. Indeed, the marital careers of the two women are virtually parallel, for Grace ultimately returns to him. However, in true Hardyian fashion, Grace's separation from her husband follows a dizzyingly sensational course. Grace seeks a divorce after Edred abandons her (true to form for a rakish scoundrel, he has run off to the Continent with a lover). Nevertheless, her attempt fails; she is not granted the divorce. Later, Edred returns to claim her, but she is unwilling to play the obedient wife. In an effort to elude him, she flees to Giles's one-room hut in the forest for help, but then faces another dilemma when inclement weather prevents Giles from taking her to a friend's house: not only do they lack a chaperone, but there is only one bed in the hut. To make matters worse, the two are not merely strangers of opposite sexes; they were formerly romantically involved. What is more, Grace has slowly fallen back in love with Giles. Thus, the idea that both might sleep in the hut cannot be countenanced, and, for three chapters, readers are witness to their dilemma: How can both halves of this would-be couple possibly find shelter with only one roof and a paralyzing host of Victorian standards of social propriety? As Grace puts it, "I am a woman, and you are a man, I cannot speak more plainly. I yearn to let you in, but—you know what is in my mind, because you know me so well."[91]

Like *Ghosts*, *The Woodlanders* becomes a novel about the bounds of social propriety at this point, for Giles insists upon sleeping outside in the cold, damp, and rain, in spite of a feverish illness. Indeed, Giles and Grace are so meticulous in their adherence to social mores that Giles situates Grace in his home "without so much as crossing the threshold himself."[92] From outside the hut, he literally locks her in, such that she is safely secreted from any male [physical] contact, including his own. From this point on, Giles signals his presence when necessary by "tapping at the window," and he communicates with Grace only through this limited opening, which (thankfully for their consciences) allows for considerably less proximity than the doorframe.[93] Though dangerously ill, Giles sleeps outside in the rain for three nights, based on the necessities mandated by social decorum, and he dies a few days later.

The text adroitly leaves ambiguous whether Giles's stint in the rain ultimately causes his death. When Grace asks Edred's professional opinion, seeking to alleviate her guilt for her complicity, Edred replies that "no human being could answer," though he adds that it is likely Giles would have died in any event, given his advanced condition.[94] Thus, while he owns that "the balance of probabilities turn[s] in her favor," he provides no definitive answer.[95] Whatever the cause of Giles's death, what matters is that the dying man suffered alone in the "damp obscurity" on the margins of Grace's cozy living space in order to protect the socially prescribed virtue of his beloved.[96]

Grace's attempts to maintain a veneer of propriety fare as miserably as Helene's. To begin with, Hardy boldly inserted the possibility of divorce into his text, a possibility that puts social and legal proprieties at odds, revealing both to be arbitrary. Although shocked by the idea, Giles accepts that "a new law might do anything," revealing both a belief in the validity of old-order customs and a blind faith in anything deemed legally acceptable.[97] When the divorce is denied, Giles reacts with predictable acceptance of the legal decree, and Giles and Grace separate, acquiescing in the mandate of both the legal law and the law of social decorum until a fit of desperation drives her back to him under less than proper circumstances. Grace's flight to Giles and away from the return of her husband causes her to begin to chafe, however fitfully, at the bonds of social decorum. She flees to Giles during a resurgence of her natural "Daphnean instinct," which has been "revived by her widowed seclusion" in Edred's absence.[98] More importantly, the narrator notes, this instinct "was not lessened by her affronted sentiments towards . . . [Fitzpiers], and her regard for another man."[99] Thus, it is not only her desire to flee from Edred but also, and more importantly, her continued (though unconsummated) passion for Giles that leads her to approach his home in the woods.

Once she arrives, though, Grace's niggling sense of propriety kicks back in, and she refuses to enter the hut, asking only for his help in traveling to a friend's house. Significantly, Giles has been ill since their last encounter, "the result of a chill caught the previous winter, seem[ing] [to have] acquire[d] virulence with the prostration of his hopes" of obtaining Grace in the only socially sanctioned manner through the potential of her divorce.[100] Thus, his illness is literally an infection contracted from adherence to the code of domestic morality, which mandates that the couple honor Grace's legal marriage, and he ultimately dies because he cannot loose himself from a commitment to social ideals. Grace, on the other hand, slowly frees herself from these fetters. Beginning with her flight to Giles's hut, her devotion to propriety begins to dissolve. When Giles, for instance, questions the decorum of her actions, Grace is firm that "appearance is no matter when the reality is right."[101]

The change, however, is slow and faltering. Most notably, although she still allows Giles to sleep outside for propriety's sake, she begins to consider the boundaries of social decorum while she herself is safe and warm in the hut. Wondering about the "rightness" of the "reality" that mandates a man sleep outside in the rain, she begins to question their setup. At one point, she asks, with "renewed misgiving," if Giles has a "snug place out there," and his answer temporarily quiets her conscience.[102] The next evening, she veers back toward appearances when she reiterates her resolution to adhere to middle-class virtue, asserting: "You know what I feel for you, but as I have vowed myself to somebody else than you . . . I must behave as I do behave, and keep that vow."[103] But soon after, she begins to have glimmers of Osvaldesque clarity, declaring, "I am not bound to [Fitzpiers] by any *divine* law after what he has done; but I have promised, and I will pay."[104] She thus simultaneously acknowledges both social mandates and her own sense of the matter—and in invoking "divine" law even asserts that God must also see things as she does. Although she remains a "ghost," as Ibsen would put it, she is beginning to inch forward from the shadows, ever braver and more confident in her ability to face the light.

As Grace grows in her sense of a personal morality, she recognizes that if Giles is suffering in his outdoor abode, "it was she who had caused it. . . . [S]he was not worth such self-sacrifice; she should not have accepted it of him."[105] With this insight, she rushes outside to look for Giles and calls for him to come in. When she receives no answer, she retreats into the house, "overpowered by her own temerity." A few minutes later, however, she rushes out again, calling loudly, *"Come to me, dearest! I don't mind what they say or what they think of us anymore."*[106] In this moment, Grace first begins to recognize the price she and Giles have paid for their commitment to conventional ideals. Shortly before his death, Grace abandons convention and drags Giles into the hut, where she undresses him, exchanges his wet clothes for dry ones, and kisses him repeatedly—thereby contracting his illness.[107] Finally, regardless of the consequences—and she recognizes that Edred's "assistance [i]s fatal to her own concealment"—she summons her husband to Giles's bedside in an effort to help revive him.[108]

While Grace ultimately learns to abandon her ties to decorum and to engage risk encounters, her initial loyalty to conventional morality has dire consequences. The "snug place" of refuge to which Giles retreats in an effort to protect Grace's reputation "prove[s] to be a wretched little shelter of the roughest kind, formed of four hurdles thatched with brake-fern"—hardly the place for an ailing man.[109] But Grace's "wish to keep the proprieties as well as [she] can" keeps her from noticing the signs of Giles's suffering. For example, "She d[oes] not notice how his hand sh[akes]," as he lights a lantern for her convenience before he leaves, and this early oversight allows for her later "erroneous conclusion" that his absences are indicative of work rather than invalidism, as well as her assumption that a "squirrel or a bird" has made the coughing noises she hears.[110] The old-order virtue they espouse most likely kills Giles and, at best, makes him suffer alone. If women cease to be signifiers of hearth and home in the system of middle-class marriage and domesticity when male-vectored disease is introduced, then Giles, in his overdetermined and insistent chivalry, ceases to signify in the text at all.[111] His body becomes a site of disease precisely because of their commitment to superficial ideals, as Grace, too, recognizes after his death: "How selfishly correct I am always—too, too correct! Can it be that cruel propriety is killing the dearest heart that ever woman clasped to her own!"[112]

Notably, both Giles and Grace act in accordance with conventional morality, revealing Hardy's and Ibsen's shared sense that *both* men and women are equally trapped, but also equally complicit, in a problematic way of defining morality and righteousness—a way of thinking that does nothing but inject disease (literally and figuratively) into the very homes, families, and societies it is intended to uphold. This is writ large in the text as Grace falls ill after Giles's death, likely from having kissed him during his illness.

This point is integral to my reading of the novel. Much to the chagrin of Hardy's contemporaries, *The Woodlanders* concludes with the reunion of Grace and her husband. Further, Edred is not only a reformed man, but he cures Grace with a "liquid . . . of a brownish hue"—even though he knows she contracted her illness from contact with Giles, and even though she has (falsely) told him that he should interpret this contact in "the extremest sense."[113] Thus, Grace's happy ending is doubly so, for her husband is willing to turn a blind eye to a supposed affair *and* to help cure her of a sexually transmitted disease. Such an ending poses a sharp contrast to the overtly bleak ending of *Ghosts*, and it struck many reviewers as glib and out of sync with their reality. Many reviewers found it neither likely nor possible for a man to forgive social transgressions such as Grace's, but many also took issue with *her* willingness to forgive *him*.[114]

To understand Hardy's ostensibly blithe ending to a story that is otherwise quite similar to *Ghosts*, it is important to consider the slow and meticulous process through which Grace and Edred reunite, a process in which each learns to leave loyalty to social decorum behind. By the time Edred reemerges on the scene with his medicine, Giles's death has already jarred Grace out of her unthinking adherence to social mores. Once she finally drags Giles back into the hut, it is too late to save him, but her paradigm shift allows her to flout convention and claim that Edred ought to make the "extremest inference" from her living situation with Giles.[115]

As for Edred, it is his willingness to figuratively inoculate himself with a dose of his own medicine via his unconditional acceptance of Grace that allows for their reunion. As elaborated in chapter 2, inoculation entails purposely injecting contaminated matter into the skin in an effort to catalyze immunity in the host and thus involves willingly accepting something threatening in the hopes of gaining ultimate resistance to it. Edred inoculates himself by subjecting himself to his own set of humiliating experiences—mirroring Grace's prior experiences—in order to strengthen their relationship. Conversely, Helene refuses to give up her commitment to propriety and inoculate herself against the debilitating effects of overdetermined social codes—for example, she won't risk appearing impious to insure the orphanage; never leaves her husband; and almost never tells her son the truth, even to protect him.

Edred's inoculation requires the complete abandonment of his allegiance to social convention and traditional gender norms. Upon his return, Edred first writes Grace, asking her to pack a suitcase and meet him at a port to leave with him, as he is unwilling to return to the site of his shame; he does not want to open himself up to public criticism or face Grace's father, who previously humiliated him.[116] But this approach only spurs her flight, as she realizes Edred "ha[s] no intention of showing himself on land at all."[117] Later, when he finally encounters her at Giles's hut, he placidly accepts her story that she has lived with Giles in the "extremest" sense, He bears witness to the scene "not so much in its intrinsic character . . . but in its character as the counterpart" of his own extramarital relationships and merely states that he does not "claim . . . any right" to her and that "it is for [her] to do and say what [she] chooses."[118] Furthermore, he is eager to help her avoid infection, even though he believes she has contracted her illness through sexual intercourse with Giles, and provides her with the medicine she needs. In doing so, he inoculates himself with his own poison, giving up his patriarchal claim to sole sexual interaction with Grace's body in a way that would have been considered particularly emasculating by contemporary standards.

As Edred progresses in his transformation, he willingly undergoes a series of humiliations. He begins by moving back into Grace's father's home, which exacts upon him at least some of the shame and stress that Grace has suffered at his hands, and he bears "all that cost . . . without flinching, because [he] . . . [feels] . . . [he] deserve[s] humiliation."[119] He becomes willing to prostrate himself entirely in the hopes of winning Grace back: "To lay offerings on her slighted altar was his first aim, and until her propitiation was complete he would constrain her in no way to return to him. . . . [H]e . . . found solace in the soft miseries she caused him."[120] In the last chapters of the novel, while living under his father-in-law's roof, Edred simply waits while allowing Grace to do as she pleases. He purposely positions himself to feel what Grace must have felt—and he revels in experiencing her prior pain by proxy. In fact, it is his very belief in her sexual affair with Giles that begins to kindle a "smouldering admiration of her" within him, as he witnesses her concomitant ability to move past propriety.[121] In the final phase of his shifting persona, Edred tells Grace that he never more "want[s] [her] to receive [him] again for duty's sake, or anything of that sort," evincing a newfound conviction that a true marriage can only exist *outside* of the constraints of the standing moral order.[122]

Ultimately, it is Edred's and Grace's parallel growth that brings them back together. Like the medicine with which Edred swoops in to save Grace's life, the effect of their mutual growth is "not miraculous . . . [but] remarkable," and the two slowly grow close, as they both learn—first separately, and then together—to ignore the bonds of propriety and act in accordance with their own sense of morality.[123] The cure is both literal and metaphoric, as it signals the release of both Grace and Edred from their blind adherence to social mores and allows for the healing of their relationship. Only then can they step forward together and face the new sun—a sun that no longer suggests a chilling mockery of conventional morality, but that harkens a new day, full of possibilities.

Enjoying Death in the Darkness:
Fin-de-Siècle Pessimism in *Jude the Obscure*

Ibsen's *Ghosts* shatters the myth that an individual or family can be immune to pervasive societal taints lurking in predominant social values. By attempting to quarantine her family via moral righteousness to set them beyond the reach of moral and physical degeneracy, Helene only guarantees their contamination. In *The Woodlanders*, Hardy presents a unique take on tainted social propriety by making flagrant subversion of hegemonic social mores the *only* social curative. By depicting a couple that could only find happiness together through complete disregard for social norms and fear of infectious disease, Hardy showed not only that valorization of purity contaminates, but also that—paradoxically—meaningful existence can only be found in the tainted spaces on the margins of moral and physical normativity.

Both Ibsen's and Hardy's texts vividly illustrate that the family that considers itself immune to the universal taint of society is in for a brutal awakening. The characters in *Ghosts* remain "abysmally afraid of the light," while those in *The Woodlanders* manage to edge their way into the pleasant glow of the "bright but heatless sun." In *Jude the Obscure* (1896), only "scintillating" glimmers of hope penetrate the bleakly obscure *fin-de-siècle* cosmology of the novel.

In *Ghosts*, the Alving family's image of moral superiority is maintained through Helene's fastidious efforts to hide her husband's lifelong habits of drunkenness and philandering. She is startled, of course, to find that, in spite of her efforts, her son has contracted syphilis due to his father's lifestyle. The family is torn apart, its theoretical golden perfection shown for the base metal that it is, and Osvald descends into catatonia, repeatedly asking his mother to give him "the sun." In *The Woodlanders*, Hardy depicts a couple who discover, through trial and error, that abandoning these ideals provides a means to happiness.

In *Jude the Obscure*, published about ten years later, Hardy complicates this idea. In the scientific and cultural milieu of the extreme end of the nineteenth century, when the ideals of the New Woman were gaining momentum and "germ hunter" bacteriologists feverishly competed to identify the next important microbe, *Jude* presents a bleaker but more complex— often nearly paradoxical—set of views. As I will show in greater detail in the next chapter, New Woman fiction provided great theoretical liberation, but practical social changes were often long in coming. The same seemed to prove true for germ theory. Its powers had been lauded in the 1870s and '80s, as it gained cultural clout for its theoretical demystification of death and disease. Yet, even as scientists gained renown for identifying microbes and bacteria, diseases such as cholera and tuberculosis remained as deadly as ever. In many ways society remained at a loss for practical solutions, in spite of a plethora of new epistemologies offering the prospect of ever-more-hopeful futures. At the turn of a new century, the one-to-one relationship between the lofty promises of science and improved realities seemed frustratingly out of step, and the literature of the period reflects this, often depicting brave new concepts, but with anticlimactic or tragic endings (Kate Chopin's *The Awakening* is a good example). In *Jude the Obscure*, everything seems tainted. Gone are the bushy sheep of Wessex, and even the acrid beauty of the heath is nowhere to be found. There are only grimy stones, misguided stonemasons, and a writhing mass of unfulfilled and unfulfilling sexual relationships.

Sue and Jude, like Grace and Edred before them, reject conventional morality. Using modern ideals inspired by a variety of progressive (albeit not always contemporary) philosophical systems, they embark upon a journey of subversion, living together and having children outside of marriage in an almost hyperbolic rejection of hegemonic norms. Further, both of them refuse to lie about their relationship, asserting that to do so would be untrue to their value system, and they both wear the hardships incurred as badges of honor even as their choices rip their family apart. Their tragic end is well known. I argue that by the time of *Jude*'s publication, Hardy complicates his original view that mere resistance to conventional ideals is sufficient to achieve positive social change. Of course, Hardy maintained in a great many of his works that society brutally punishes nonnormative behaviors. But more is at stake in *Jude the Obscure*. First, the novel shows that Sue and Jude's unconventional morals, when they espouse them, exhibit the same separatism of moral righteousness as the status quo. Sue and Jude often nearly catch glimpses of this reality themselves, as their own inconsistent behaviors and shifting values famously indicate. In *Jude the Obscure*, Hardy depicts characters who tiptoe at the edge of flouting social norms, dallying momentarily just past its bounds and then frantically retreating to the safety of hegemonic norms, again and again. What I want to focus on in this chapter, however, are the ways in which Jude and Sue's moments of nonconformity, when they appear, are cloaked in all the moral superiority that the status quo itself invokes to enforce more commonly held beliefs (such as matrimonial sanctity and purity). A few brief examples ought to suffice to indicate this, as the characters' very caprices result in their inhabiting unconventional stances only briefly at any given time. In fact, Hardy was honing a more insistent discussion on catalyzing broad social changes via unconventional lifestyles, a subject that I will address further in the next chapter.

For all her belief in the superiority of her unmarried life with Jude, Sue's words mirror conventional moralizing tones when she scolds Jude for returning to Arabella for a sexual encounter after their separation:

> How will the demi-gods in your Pantheon—I mean those legendary persons you call Saints—intercede for you after this? Now if *I* had done such a thing it would have been different, and not remarkable, for at least I don't regard marriage as a sacrament.[124]

For Jude's part, while his lofty educational aims began as a real hunger for knowledge, they are later depicted as having fossilized into mere habit and social ambition when he decides early on to abandon university for the lay ministry:

> The old fancy which had led on to the culminating vision of the bishopric had not been an ethical or theological enthusiasm at all, but a mundane ambition masquerading in a surplice. He feared that his whole scheme had degenerated to, even though it might not have originated in, a social unrest which had no foundation in the nobler instincts; which was purely an artificial product of civilization.[125]

In their lowest moments, Sue and Jude (unlike Grace and Edred) do not truly accept one another outside of moral norms. Rather, in their vacillations between value systems, the moments where they embrace subversions seem to demonstrate only more of the same moralizing that characterizes broader social norms, only aimed at different ends. In depicting their motives this way, Hardy suggests that Sue and Jude are no better than Helene; although they may reject the status quo, their divergent path tends toward the same ends of self-preservation and the isolated superiority of moral righteousness.

To some extent, *Jude*'s complexities can be linked to the late-century attitudes outlined above: like many authors at the century's close, Hardy exhibits an increasing lack of faith (typical at the very end of the century) in the power of progressive ideals to create a new and improved reality. But I would also like to suggest that Hardy cast Sue and Jude as participants in an unconventional lifestyle for purely conventional ends. While Grace and Edred learn to grow together and realize they can do so only outside of moral orthodoxy, Sue and Jude each use conventionally moralistic pretenses in their pursuit of subversion *as* moral righteousness—something Hardy casts as an equally degenerative tactic. As Jude unwittingly notes, to "do an immoral thing for moral reasons" is a rather paltry ethical defense.[126]

Ultimately, it is Little Father Time who ushers in the beginning of the end for Sue and Jude. And it is through him that Hardy vividly shows that no one, no matter how advanced or subversive, is immune to the effects of decades of broad moral contamination. Like Ibsen, Hardy demonstrates in *Jude* that those who buy into the delusion of personal salvation in a vacuum of moral purity, quarantined from their fellow men, will fairly quickly hear their own figurative—and often literal—death knell. Disillusionment with progressive ideals in this period contributed in some obvious ways, therefore, to the development of this fictional outcome. Hardy's ethical meliorism, a sort of moral evolution that developed alongside his work, likely also contributed to this fictional-philosophical dénouement. If, as Hardy argued, attaining the best of the world "exacts a full look at its worst," his view of ethical meliorism involved a precursorial, ritualized cleansing in which society, at all extremes, was forced to recognize its mutual interdependence by accepting the byproducts of its own social diseases. *Jude the Obscure* loudly proclaims, in its characteristically sermonic style, that no one is immune or quarantined in a globalized, interpersonal world and that no one can circumvent the consequences of self-contamination. It is Little Father Time who visits this truth upon Jude, Sue, and their family.

The child, though only about eight years old, appears shriveled and aged. He has an "octogenarian face," and is "Age masquerading as Juvenility, and doing it so badly that his real self showed through crevices."[127] As he travels ominously on a train bound for Jude and his family equipped with only a key and a ticket (highly symbolic possessions), the narrator describes him as "a ground swell from ancient years of night," an "aged child," and a "singular child" with a "quaint and weird face."[128] Children born with syphilis contracted in utero were described by contemporary medical accounts using much the same language. "This *look of little old men,* so common in new-born children doomed to syphilis" was acknowledged by most medical professionals to be one of the most characteristic signs of congenital syphilis.[129] Going into greater detail, Fournier describes syphilitic infants thusly in his 1882 *Syphilis and Marriage*:

> They come into the world small, singularly weak and puny, poorly developed, wrinkled and shriveled, stunted, with the "old man look," as it is usually termed. One would call them old people in miniature, with a skin too large for them over certain points. . . . Nothing else . . . of a special character attests a well-pronounced syphilitic state in . . . these little old people, as they are called. . . . And, nevertheless, at the first glance, one judges correctly that they will not live. . . . These children do not die, properly speaking; they fade out rather than die; they cease to live, for the sole reason that they are not viable, that they are unequal to life.[130]

Another late-century medical text affirms these general assessments of the syphilitic child:

> The child often looks prematurely aged; its hair may have fallen off, even the eyelashes and from the eyebrows; the corners of the lips and nose are often ulcerated. . . . Progressive and general emaciation is a very unfavorable sign, the skin becoming of a dirty white, and hanging from the muscles, which are soft. In taking up a fold of the skin it is found to be inelastic, cold, and harsh.[131]

Contemporary medical texts were not lacking for detailed illustrations of such children, either (see Figures 4.1 and 4.2).[132] From the description

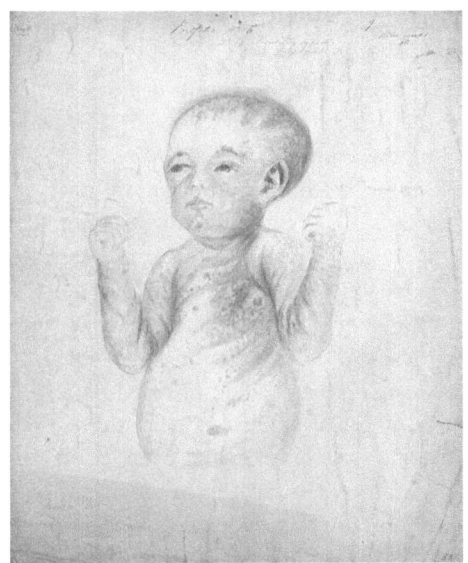

Figures 4.1. Illustration of Infant with Congenital Syphilis, 1856.

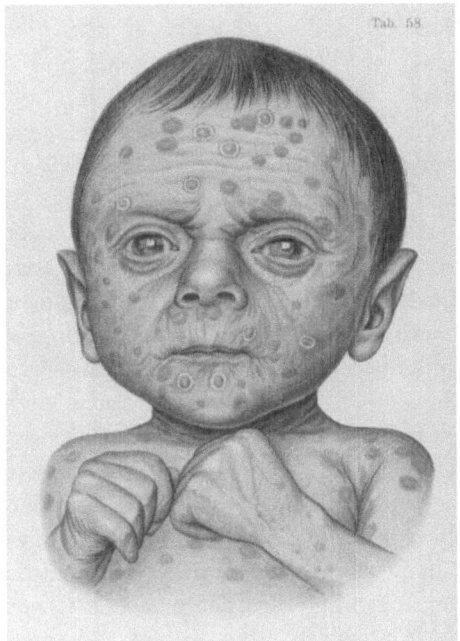

Figure 4.2. Illustration of Infant with Congenital Syphilis, 1898.

of Little Father Time's "quaint and weird face," with skin loose and sagging "like the tragic mask of Melpomene," to the doctor's assessment of his death, which indicates that "such boys are springing up. . . . they . . . see all its [life's] terrors before they are old enough to have . . . staying power. . . . [they are] the beginning of the coming universal wish not to live," Little Father Time's tale evokes syphilitic children in the late part of the century.[133] It is no great leap, given Hardy's engagement with popular science, to read Little Father Time as an equally medically accurate rendering of a syphilitic child as Osvald is as a syphilitic adult. Hardy made it easy for readers to doubt Arabella's constancy to Jude, so paired with her flight to Australia—a place saturated with the symbolic ethos of criminals and criminality in the Victorian era—and Little Father Time's physical description, contemporary readers could infer a microbial subtext in the novel in which Arabella contracts syphilis in Australia while pregnant with Jude's child.[134]

In *Ghosts*, an estranged son born from a conventional marriage returns to deconstruct the normative family who has attempted in vain to avoid risk encounters; the dynamic that *Jude* depicts goes farther, revealing that even "advanced" moral systems are no protection against the universal taint of conventional morality. Society must reap what it has sown before the social fields can lie fallow and nourish new growth. As Jude laments after the death of his children, "Things are as they are, and will be brought to their destined issue."[135]

Thus, if the characters in *Ghosts* hide as they "glide . . . between the lines" of the letter of the social law, while *The Woodlanders'* Grace and Edred manage to find their way into a pleasant, sunny grove, Sue and Jude must effectively live out the Browning epigraph that introduces the tragically climactic final book of their story: "There are two who decline, a woman and I, / And enjoy our death in darkness here."[136] Though it is their arrogant attempt at moral martyrdom that in many ways brings about their doom, Hardy effectively martyred them to a different cause—they are the evolutionary products of a society based on worm-eaten ideals. This soil must, as Hardy shows, putrefy before it can leave room for new growth. In this way, literal and figurative disease is in fact the only potential regenerative fertilizer in the moral desert of the 1890s. This injection of literal disease forces even the self-righteous Jude and Sue to recognize that isolated asepsis is an impossibility in an interdependent society. Little Father Time is the key and the ticket to understanding their doom, as it is his congenitally diseased body that unravels their selfish moral system and forces them to accept their necessary involvement in the world around them. As Sue says when

Little Father Time comes into their lives, "I feel myself getting intertwined with my kind."[137] Thus, it is only through their final tentative embrace of infectious disease, in a brief scene that has been given little critical attention, that Hardy showed that salvation in a secularized world lies in contaminated pathways that highlight the inescapable interdependence of humanity.

"A Chaos of Principles—Groping in the Dark"

Little Father Time, with his "octogenarian" face "singularly deficient in all the usual hopes of childhood," most obviously represents the conventional ideals of Jude's legal (and thereby supposedly ethical and natural) marriage coming back to wreak havoc on the literally natural and extralegal family he has constructed.[138] He is the return of the repressed, embodied in a ghostly, waifish, sick child. But he signifies still more. He also highlights the inescapable universal taint of the time, where so-called advanced ideals were insufficient to combat the leavings of previous ideologies. Indeed, as Jude expounds upon his sense of "groping in the dark," late in the novel, "I perceive there is something wrong somewhere in our social formulas: what it is can only be discovered by men or women with greater insight than mine."[139] Little Father Time is—figuratively and literally—the Reaper, come to display the (rotten) fruits of Sue and Jude's moral toils and to insist that *all* of society must reap what it has sown. As he eerily whispers to his parents near the novel's conclusion, "It do seem like Judgment Day!"[140] He represents, therefore, the "chaos of principles" that Jude describes upon his return to Christminster. He embodies and enacts the force of the liminal ethical space in which *fin-de-siècle* society found itself—shuffling hesitatingly past older order Victorian values of the hearth and home, but only toward a hazy precipice where deterministic gravitational laws dwarfed theoretical moral principles. At times, the narrator overtly plays on Little Father Time's embodiment of this liminal conceptual world: " 'Where do we go to?' asked Time, in suspense."[141] He is time embodied and suspended, hanging between two worlds, a pendulum paused in the upswing. As such, he is "doubly awake, like an enslaved and dwarfed Divinity, sitting passive and regarding his companions as if he saw their whole rounded lives rather than their immediate figures."[142]

It is, of course, because of a misunderstanding—or, one could argue, a too precise understanding—of Malthusian doctrines that Little Father Time kills himself and his siblings, or so most traditional readings of *Jude* would have it. His perfunctory suicide note, after all, reads simply, "Done because we are too menny," suggesting that he has taken Sue's acknowledgment that their family is too large very much to heart in his final acts.[143] Representing as he does this liminal space between two epistemologies—a liminal space that becomes a gaping hole—there is another way of reading his last words. That is, his seemingly innocuous misspelling of "many" must be seen as also a reference to the humanity or humanness of the family and their ideals.

As Talia Schaffer and Sally Shuttleworth, among others have noted, Little Father Time is the "nodal point" of Jude and Sue's story.[144] This moment is key for my reading. In physics, a "nodal point" is a moment of complete rest in an otherwise dynamic wave pattern, or a point on a sphere with the value of zero. Little Father Time is indeed the nodal point upon which the whole novel unravels. He un*does* all the *doings* of the novel. All the children are unborn, as it were, and Sue and Jude go back to their previous lives—Sue to an outwardly orthodox and zealous Christianity, and Jude to Arabella. As with Ibsen's *Ghosts*, in *Jude*, Hardy seemed to suggest that society would have been better off had all of this simply never been— that is, if society had not in fact required such a nodal point to reset the clock, to purify a contaminated society, to make way for the new generations that Sue seems so sure will come to "feel as we do" in "fifty, a hundred, years."[145] "I ought not to be born, ought I?" asks poor Little Father Time shortly before his death, and Hardy's Jeremiadic answer is "yes."[146] Jude himself unwittingly prophesies his son's death earlier when he quotes Job as he contemplates him: " 'Let the day perish wherein I was born, and the night in which it was said, there is a manchild conceived!' That's what the boy—*my* boy, perhaps, will find himself saying before long!"[147] As Little Father Time hangs in the closet alongside his siblings, making one of a "triplet of corpses," the narrator notes that:

> The boy's face expressed the whole tale of their situation. On that little shape had converged all the inauspiciousness and shadow which had darkened the first union of Jude, and all the accidents, mistakes, fears, errors of the last. He was their nodal point, their focus, their expression in a single term. For the rashness of those parents he had groaned, for their ill-assortment he had quaked, and for the misfortunes of these he had died.[148]

Like Ibsen, Hardy created a text that he paradoxically insists would be better off *not* existing, but, unlike Ibsen, he nevertheless suspends his condemnation of the two principal characters in this sequence of unworthy events. As the nodal point that unravels the novel, Little Father Time's pathetic scribble, "we are too menny," rather insists that we, like Jude and Sue, are all simply too human—too human to continue our own evolutionary success.[149] *Jude the Obscure* incorporates one of Hardy's famous poetic sentiments about a thoughtless, watchmaker-God: "At the framing of the terrestrial conditions there seemed never to have been contemplated such a development of emotional perceptiveness among the creatures subject to those conditions as that reached by thinking and educated humanity."[150]

Where society fails, we all fail. As Jude says of Little Father Time, "All the little ones of our time are collectively the children of us adults of the time, and entitled to" (or, as the narrative suggests, yoked under) "our general care."[151] No matter the ethical system—normative or subversive—no one can exist in a state of isolated success where society at large is floundering. Jude continues, acknowledging this fact even as he remains blind to its personal relevance: "The excessive regard of parents for their own children, and their dislike of other people's, is, like class-feeling, patriotism, and save-your-own-soul-ism, and other virtues, a mean exclusiveness at bottom."[152]

Let That Day Be Darkness

The only chinks of sunlight that pierce the gloomy ending of *Jude the Obscure* occur when Jude and Sue briefly accept that their fates are intertwined with that of society. Hardy, aware that the hermetically sealed sickroom is an illusion and that no one can effect any progressive change upon society from the sequestration of self-righteous ethics, sends Jude forth from the sickroom to confront Sue's aggressive moralism. By engaging in infectious intimate contact, they open themselves to deeper subjective experience and lay aside their attempts at moral or physical quarantine and asepsis.

Near the end of the novel, Jude leaves his sickroom (and eventual deathbed) and travels to confront the naively zealous Sue with his diseased and dying body, which is ravaged by tuberculosis. The text makes this fairly clear by indicating his slow decline over several months, coupled with a cough. As noted in chapter 4, tuberculosis was one of the most prevalent diseases of the day, and one of the few severe respiratory illnesses that is fatal but slow. His "ghastly pale" face marks him as consumptive even further, as the whiteness of tuberculosis patients was widely recognized at the time.[153]

Throughout the novel, Sue has marginalized Jude, always claiming the moral high road, whether through modernized reasoning and gender views or rigorous adherence to conventional Christian morality. But, far from allowing Jude to languish in the sickroom because of his marginality, Hardy explodes the space of the sickroom when Jude leaves it and confronts Sue with the very marginality she has imposed upon him, marginality that is now written upon his body in the form of fatal illness. Jude calls her to task for her superficial modes of morality, which have plagued them from the beginning:

> Is it that you are humbugging yourself, as so many women do about these things; and don't actually believe what you pretend to, and are only indulging in the luxury of the emotion raised by an affected belief? . . . You dear, sad, soft, most melancholy wreck of a promising human intellect that it has ever been my lot to behold. Where is your scorn of convention gone?[154]

As Jude confronts Sue with the fragile mess that conventional and unconventional ideologies alike have made, he momentarily changes her heart and strips her of her superficial conventionality:

> "I can't endure you to say that," she burst out, and her eye resting on him a moment, she turned back impulsively. "Don't, don't scorn me! Kiss me, o kiss me lots of times, and say I am not a coward and a contemptible humbug—I can't bear it!" She rushed up to him and, with her mouth on his, continued: "I must tell you—O I must—my darling Love! It has been—only a church marriage—an apparent marriage I mean!"[155]

Confronted with the truth that Jude's body speaks through its disease, Sue and Jude are able to move past the overdetermined moral systems that have unraveled their lives. In the face of his dying body, Sue can admit that her marriage to another man "on the altar of what she was pleased to call her principles" has not been consummated (that is, that her newest moral outfit is threadbare). More importantly, she can own her own true self by sloughing off her assumed impermeability and kissing the contagious and dying man.[156] Published in 1895, *Jude* is much too late a text for Hardy to have been unaware of the epidemiological implications of "bruising . . . with kisses" a man clearly dying of tuberculosis—and this is precisely the point.[157] By physically uniting, Sue and Jude are able to attain true interpersonal human intimacy for a moment, as they are both finally aware of the inextricably intertwined nature of all humanity.

Of course, *Jude* remains a tragedy, and the tragedy of this scene is that, after their passionate kisses, Sue retreats to the moral systems that seem to offer her safety in purity, and she returns to her "apparent marriage" to consummate it. She is "creed-drunk," much as Jude was "gin-drunk" during his marriage to Arabella, and, as Jude aptly notes during his last journey into the world of "creation's groans," "either form of intoxication takes away the nobler vision."[158] Too entrenched in her belief in the potential of isolated moral righteousness, Sue leaves Jude to return to his sickroom, in spite of his pleas: "Don't abandon me, Sue, to save your own soul only!"[159] She thus abjures the only chance they have to be together in truth and unity and abandons her chance of true self-actualization and unity with humanity. In the end, Jude returns to his sickroom to die, as Sue listens to the departing sound of "his coughs mingling with the rain on the windows."[160] The novel ends with Jude back in the sickroom, sequestered again, as he recites the lines he believed would apply only to his son, but now realizes apply to the whole of a diseased society: " 'Let the day perish wherein I was born, and the night in which it was said, There is a man child conceived. . . . Let that day be darkness . . . neither let the light shine upon it.' "[161] With nothing left certain but the certainty of a tainted society with impure morals, *Jude the Obscure* ends bleakly, its characters having but uncertainly and rather haphazardly attempted to flout the systems of norms that guided their world. By using only the tools of the system itself (that is, moral high-horsing), their efforts falter from the beginning, and are only weakly sustained at any given moment. In the next chapter, Hardy and another late-century novelist, Grant Allen, up the ante with depictions of sustained subversion in two fictional case studies of free love.

Humanity's Waste

Typhoid Fever, the Failure of Isolation, and the Development of Probiotics in Three Late-Century Works

It is the clear knowledge of the evils arising from harbouring decompos-
ing matter in the vicinity of our dwellings that has called forth, within
the last quarter of a century, certain legislative measures, the objects
of which have been to give powers to the local authorities to suppress
the evils arising from cesspools and other abominations.

—*Purification and Utilisation of Sewage,* 1876

DR. STOCKMANN: I have already told you that what I want to speak
about is the great discovery I have made lately—the discovery that all
the sources of our moral life are poisoned and that the whole fabric of
our civic community is founded on the pestiferous soil of falsehood.

—*An Enemy of the People,* 1882

Connectivity in an Age of Isolation

In this final chapter, I focus on a set of texts whose plots hinge solely on
the concept and value of isolation that I have discussed throughout this
book. In this collection, however, authors hone and shape their depictions
of what effective resistance to such hegemonic norms might look like. As
a set, they quite directly build upon the concerns played out by the works
in the previous chapter (i.e., that society as a whole is diseased, particularly

through and because of its efforts to appear pure and moral). Significantly, in so doing, the texts in this chapter depict characters who attempt to eschew this status quo through the same moral separatism they hope to resist.[1] The main characters in the texts at hand construct for themselves spaces of reactionary, countercultural moral isolation. Moreover, the authors of these works drive their point home even farther by illustrating the abject failure of these protagonists whose moral separatism—righteous or not—results in their deaths and/or destruction. No matter the cause, then, these authors suggest, individualistic practices that fail to consider the common good can never succeed; even progress must be communal. To make their points, these authors incorporate typhoid fever and discussions of sewage and waste disposal into the fiction and drama covered in this chapter.

In this chapter, I will show that Henrik Ibsen and New Woman novelist Grant Allen act with such commitment to this idea that they destroy their own main characters to demonstrate that moral separatism can never succeed. To conclude, I will highlight an odd, oft-reviled Hardy novel as a surprising illustration of openness and connectivity. I have mentioned that these texts develop the concerns laid out in the previous chapter; this is because two of the three texts I cover here are later works by the same authors and, in both cases, are the works they produced *immediately after* penning the works covered in chapter 4. The third text I cover here represents a separate author, Grant Allen, whose work, explicitly of the New Woman genre of *fin-de-siècle,* necessarily addresses the ideas about disease and bacteria developed earlier in the century, in addition to its concern with the role of social mores in shaping the individual constituents of collective society.

This chapter will cover three texts, then: Grant Allen's 1895 *The Woman Who Did,* Henrik Ibsen's 1883 *An Enemy of the People* (written one year after he wrote *Ghosts*), and Thomas Hardy's *The Well-Beloved* (written first in 1892, and then rewritten in 1897, thus uniquely bookending Hardy's problematizing of Sue and Jude's resistance portrayed in *Jude the Obscure*). In *The Woman Who Did* and *An Enemy of the People,* I will demonstrate that the authors shift the focus of their arguments and showcase individuals who attempt to rise above the diseased cesspool of society by standing alone against it—and both do so through contemporary discourse on cesspools alongside depictions of characters who attempt (and fail) to stand alone against the status quo with a like measure of countercultural moral isolationism. Both of their vivid portrayals viscerally and movingly illustrate the utter failure of such isolated resistance, highlighting the universal applicability of authorial claims against self-interested isolation, even in the form of resistance to problematic norms and practices. That is, not only do these works demonstrate the problems with germ theory's isolationist quarantine models of human existence, they transmogrify, in this later period, to include *even* like-minded, countercultural constituents into their discussions. Even in their acts of resistance, then, these authors highlight community and connection, signaling that no one person can stand alone meaningfully against the community of which they are a part. Rather, change must take place through connection with others and in conjunction with the community itself. Movement, perhaps, can be grassroots and individualized initially, but fulfilling and meaningful change must ultimately be located in communal efforts and visions. I conclude the chapter with Thomas Hardy's novel *The Well-Beloved*, which, I will show, highlights flow and connection over isolation through imagery depicted by way of actual pipelines and sewage flow—aligning itself thereby with the proto-probiotic movements of the late century. I will argue that these proto-probiotic gestures in culture and literature were the beginnings of growing acceptance of the vitalizing nature of risk and connection gaining momentum after decades of ideological emphasis on isolation and self-preservation in the wake of germ theory. These specific discussions on probiotics in sewage came out of rampant typhoid infections caused by such sewage—fevers that are encapsulated into the texts discussed here as they grapple with social change, community, and isolation.

Moral Separatism as Abiotic in Grant Allen's *The Woman Who Did*

Grant Allen's 1895 *The Woman Who Did* is, on the surface, a straightforward, arguably pedantic novella about Herminia Barton's quest to pursue free love in defiance of Victorian social mores. More specifically, she believes it is her mission in life to change society by living monogamously with her partner outside of the guises of marriage (the echoes of Sue and Jude's determination here are clear). Indeed, Hardy's *Jude the Obscure* began in serialized format in December 1894, while *The Woman Who Did* was published early in 1895. Hardy read *The Woman Who Did* while the early issues of *Jude* were still being published. He loved the book, and wrote to Allen to thank him for writing it.[2] As William Davis notes, in this letter, Hardy himself "added that it 'was curious to find how exactly [Allen] had anticipated my view.' "[3] As Hardy's earliest version of the novel was significantly bowdlerized, it may have appeared, in print at least, that Allen's concerns predated Hardy's. Regardless, the two novels appeared nearly simultaneously in print, and they spoke to similar concerns in tandem such that Spectator grouped them together as jointly promoting a repulsive "new morality."[4] Given the similarities with *Jude the Obscure,* the parallels between the two novels regarding moral isolation should be readily apparent. This is even more so because Grant Allen lends Herminia's aims a more overtly self-righteous tone than even *Jude the Obscure*'s heavy-handed moralizing. "It never occurred to me to think," Herminia tells her eventual partner, Alan Merrick, as they discuss her desire to live together without marrying, " 'my life could ever end in anything else but martyrdom. It *must* needs be so with all true lives and all good ones.'"[5] In one breath, Herminia likens herself to martyred saints, calling her own mode of living a "creed," and also claims that anyone who is not martyred is incapable of goodness.[6] When Alan accepts her terms of endearment, she expounds about her philosophy of isolated moral superiority:

> Brave women before me have tried for awhile to act . . . for the good of their sex; but never of their own free will from the very beginning. They have avoided marriage, not because they thought it a shame and a surrender, a treason to their sex . . . but because there existed at the time some obstacle in their way in the shape of the vested interested of some other woman. . . . Now, *I* have the rare chance of acting otherwise; I can show the world from the very first that I act from principle, and from principle only. . . . No other [woman] has voluntarily risen as I propose to do.[7]

Based on early feminist principles though it may be, it's hard to imagine a more egocentric speech than this. Herminia wants to flout the status quo, yes, but she aims to do so by envisioning herself as better than every woman who has ever existed in the history of the earth besides herself. While intersectional feminism and the claims of bell hooks and the like against white feminism would be decades in the making, I find it hard to imagine that even Victorian-era New Women would have found Herminia's sentiments palatable. Indeed, whether they promoted or panned the novel, critics took issue with Herminia's self-aggrandizing sense of her own moral martyrdom. H. G. Wells mocked her, in spite of concluding that the book itself was worth reading: "Her soul is 'spotless.' Never did she do anything wrong. (And this is a 'real woman'!)."[8] Another more sympathetic review also recommended the book, but warned that Herminia was "at times . . . too dogmatic for ordinary mortals."[9] A more negative review by Millicent Garrett Fawcett nevertheless agreed upon this assessment of Herminia as character, complaining that the " 'spotless woman's' moral grandeur is insisted upon *ad nauseum*."[10] Continuing on about Herminia's irksome "saintlike attitude" (an epithet that is decidedly not intended as a compliment), Fawcett ridicules Herminia's moral superiority in thought and depiction:

> She . . . [is] not . . . afflicted with any of the ills that flesh is heir to, not having, for instance, washing bills like a *mere* woman, she dressed in pure white from head to foot. She is not eager to be happy . . . but "sets out in life with the earnest determination to be a martyr," keeping prussic acid as a last resort if the process of martyrdom becomes uncomfortable. She converses in set speeches several pages in length, and she repeats with tiresome iteration on every alternate page or so, that she is the *one woman in the whole world* who is really free. . . . She talks pages about her "higher longings" and the "yearnings" peculiar to her about the degradation of other women and *her own vast superiority*.[11]

Decrying the character-messenger separate from the message, contemporary reviews of *The Woman Who Did*, whether positive or negative, clearly indicate that Herminia's approach to her philosophy was judged differently from the philosophy itself. Particularly in the more positive reviews, we can glean a clear sense of Allen's insistence that the ends do not justify the means of isolationist practice and thinking. Moreover, it is clear that his readers clearly and rather uniformly cited her moral superiority as her fatal flaw, regardless of their stance on her actual acts of resistance. "Its purpose is everything," an appreciative reviewer notes, while adding in the same sentence that "its people [are] nothing." The same reviewer continues on, arguing that while "his remedy will, no doubt, seem to many worse than the disease; yet no one but a fool can fail to admit the disease."[12]

Although the reviewer here ascribes the remedy to Allen, I would argue that the language of the reviews overall criticizes *Herminia's* approach, separate from their assessments of the absence or presence of a social disease in Victorian marriage norms. Thus, I would argue that the remedy is Herminia's, not necessarily Allen's, particularly insofar as Herminia is killed off at the end of the story. Critics and reviewers have, in fact, never been sure what to make of Allen's ending because of its very tendency to cast his otherwise countercultural novel into the genre of fallen-woman fiction.

Wouldn't this ending rather serve as a warning *against* her actions, like any stereotypical fallen woman plot? The best explanation for this dissonance is to separate, as the Victorians obviously did, Herminia's choice of remedy *within* the book from Allen's authorial act of writing the book itself as a formal diagnosis of this disease. She dies as a warning, yes, but no reader of this explicitly and pedantically earnest New Woman novel could interpret this as an admonition to embrace the "disease" of Victorian marriage norms that the entire novel cries out against. It is possible to see her death as mere tragedy—the sacrifice of an innocent amid an unforgiving world—but if we take seriously the wide berth of Victorian reviewers who said, in one form or another, that the disease may have existed, but her remedy was problematic, it is possible to see her failure as the very isolationist thinking that enables her to believe that she is morally superior to other women, and thus solely and uniquely capable of saving the entire sex alone. In fact, this isolation is no mere byproduct of her life, but an integral part of her disease "remedy."

As I've mentioned, Allen's novel develops the concerns highlighted in *Jude the Obscure* (that of an inherently diseased society rotting away because of its own moral hang-ups). The two novels handle disease somewhat differently, however. That is, Allen's novel attempts to envision what effective and ineffective resistance to this society might look like. The rhetoric of contamination undergirds the explicitly feminist aims of the novel, in spite of the plot having very little to do with disease. While there is one death by actual disease in the novel (of which more later), actual incurred illness is largely discursively substituted with fears of contamination. Allen deftly extrapolates common post-germ-theory concerns about disease into the metaphoric potential of these fears as he illustrates the common human tendency to tend toward self-righteous isolation that sees anything outside the self as noxious and disordered. He virtually anticipates and pairs, thereby, the Kristevan notions of the I/not-I abject and Mary Douglas's famous discourse on impurity as that which is labeled out of systemic order. Here, Grant marries the psychological heft of Kristeva's and Douglas's theories to demonstrate that there is no natural abject; rather, humans abject*ify* one another in an attempt to preserve the personal subject's order.

Crucially, in the novel, while these moments often occur predictably when characters representing the Victorian status quo criticize Herminia, they equally as often are Herminia's own language, speaking of the contaminating influences *of* the status quo. The voices of the moral hegemony unsurprisingly discuss the possibility of Herminia's contaminating influence on other women. "You are not fit to receive a pure girl's kisses," Dolly shouts at her mother before leaving her for the last time, and her final words echo the predictable Victorian language of sexual impropriety with contamination.[13] More unexpected is Herminia's casting of the same rhetorical stones back at the hegemonic majority. She invokes the notion of filthy or contaminated lucre by refusing to join her estates with Alan, refusing to taint their relationship with "any sordid stain or money, any vile tinge of bargaining."[14] Later, after Alan's death, his father travels to Italy to see the two, and offers Herminia money. She frantically shouts at him, "Don't pollute my table!" and demands that he take it back.[15] The narrator joins in her rhetoric after her return to England with her daughter, commenting on the "leprous taint" of the status quo.[16] Perhaps most powerful, however, is the scene early in the novel in which Alan's father disowns him, saying "in a chilly voice" that he "must guard [his] mother and sisters . . . from the contamination of this woman's opinions,"[17] which is neatly counterbalanced against one much later in the novel in which the same man gives Herminia's daughter money, knowing that Herminia is struggling to make ends meet. When she sees the coin, Herminia "ca[tches] her child up with a cry of terror," and then "change[s] the tainted sovereign . . . for another one."[18] If Herminia's motives here were not clear enough, the narrator immediately adds that "the child who was born to free half the human race from aeons of slavery must be kept from all contagion of man's gold and man's bribery."[19]

This phrase is in fact the source for the title of this book. And it is, I hope, clear by now that I believe many authors in this period strove to indicate that no one—whether born to free the human race or not—can ever be fully or profitably "kept from all contagion" issuing from their fellow humans. To use Herminia's own words, *The Woman Who Did* stands as an antithesis to the idea that anyone can survive by setting their individual "hearts against the world" and ignoring that social world of which they are necessarily a part.[20]

Here are obvious connections, then, to Hardy's and Ibsen's works in the previous chapter where the two authors invert the hegemonic language of purity and contamination to affirm their own arguments about the internal disease of Victorian purity itself. Allen counterposes these two viewpoints (which he embodies in sets of characters scrambling to identify each other as impure, however) and shifts the focus from that of the texts in chapter 4. Here, instead of an interesting subversion-via-inversion of claims to purity and contamination, Allen rather demonstrates that *anyone* in power will attempt to castigate an other as impure, while holding him- or herself as situated in the isolated purity of moral superiority. As Douglas has so famously explicated, ritual uncleanness and secular hygiene are essentially one and the same. As she puts it:

> If we can abstract pathogenicity and hygiene from our notion of dirt, we are left with the old definition of dirt as matter out of place . . . where there is dirt there is system. Dirt is the by-product of a systematic ordering and classification of matter, in so far as ordering involves rejecting inappropriate elements. The idea of dirt takes us straight into the field of symbolism and promises a link-up with more obviously symbolic systems of purity. We can recognize in our own notions of dirt that we are using a kind of omnibus compendium which includes all the rejected elements of ordered systems. It is a relative idea.[21]

Allen's juxtaposition, then, of sets of parties accusing each other of contamination reveals the self-interested nature of any and all claims to purity. He demonstrates this inclination to be misguided and subject to fail through Herminia's eventual downfall. By paralleling both his countercultural protagonist and the voices of the hegemonic majority in their shared desire to reify hierarchies of purity and righteousness, Allen castigates both.

After living monogamously, but unmarried with her partner, and separating herself from a society she views as contaminating, she loses Alan to typhoid fever, and ultimately loses even her daughter's love and dies alone—via suicide. At the conclusion of the novel, Dolly revolts against what she admittedly correctly sees as her mother's stifling exploitation of her for her own philosophical ends. To the end, Herminia maintains an egocentric view of the matter, even in her grief. She is shocked that "the child predestined" in her own grandiose imaginings "to regenerate humanity, was thinking for herself."[22] With polemics set as Herminia has constructed them, Dolly has no real method of revolt except to veer to the other extreme of society and incorporate herself into the status quo. Herminia kills herself after Dolly leaves her for a traditional, lucrative marriage. Herminia's death certainly signals the failure of the method by which she has attempted to facilitate social progress. Her belief in purity via isolation is proven thereby to be patently false. Moreover, her death by suicide indicates even further the *de*vitalizing nature of this means of attaining purity. Just like the examples illustrated by all of the previous authors covered in this book, Allen shows isolated safety—whether from contaminating morals or contaminating pathogens—to be unsustainable. Life will simply not thrive in aseptic purity, which he reveals, like the authors covered here before him, to be antibiotic—opposed to life.

The ultimate and unmistakable failure of her experiment works in tandem with her defensive assertions that not only is the status quo impure but that she (alone) *is* pure, to demonstrate Allen's aims that a meaningful life cannot be fulfilled in isolation. Make no mistake—just as earlier authors' depictions of the futility of risk-averse quarantine does *not* imply their endorsement of intentional martyrdom and death via voluntarily acquired infection, here, too, we have a similar reversal of a reversal. This ideology doubles back on itself—Allen (and Ibsen and Hardy) pronounces that social progress against and beyond the status quo cannot occur through the same self-congratulatory, morally isolated route of superiority the status quo itself is built upon. This does not, however, mean that these authors advocated acceptance of the status quo. For one, any cursory reading of Ibsen's or Hardy's works, or that of the New Woman writers, is evidence of this. More to the point: these authors, in imagining what progressive social and moral solutions might look like, warn against the same sort of extremism the status quo grounded itself in to begin with. There may be social and moral diseases to cleanse, indeed, but as Allen's narrator admonishes in finely rendered scientific prose, "no unit can wholly sever itself from the social organism of which it is a corpuscle."[23]

The fact that Herminia's partner, Alan Merrick, dies early in the novel of typhoid fever is a key component to Grant Allen's claims about isolationist purity. Its presence is even more notable because typhoid is a disease not typically named outright in Victorian texts, due to its associations with the indelicacies of fecal matter and bodily excretions. In fact, not only is the disease mentioned—a rarity in itself—but it is described precisely as a pathogen linking humans to one another and to their environment. As a "filth disease," Victorians readily accepted that typhoid was caused by human waste and contact with it.[24] Allen incorporates these understandings into his discussion of the days leading up to Alan's death, describing Herminia's disgust with the town of Perugia, full, as she sees it, of "devouring wastes of rubbish and foul . . . kitchen-middens [refuse piles]."[25] Ironically, however, though Alan dies in Perugia, the doctor and narrator both note that he acquired his infection in Florence (which Herminia thinks of as a "dream of delight," and "*pure* gold"), once again signaling the misguided aims of Herminia's predilections.[26] Not the least of her misperceptions here includes her disgust with the "odours" of Perugia, which codes her as outdated in her espousal of the older-order miasma theory, while she remains completely ignorant of the real danger in seemingly pure Florentine water.[27]

In Perugia, the doctor pronounces his case. "This is typhoid fever," he determines, "a very bad type."[28] The omniscient narrator confirms the pathogenic identification here, again affirming Herminia's mistaken approach to the world:

> He spoke the plain truth. Twenty-one days before, in his bed-room at the hotel in Florence, Alan had drunk a single glass of water from the polluted springs that supply in part the Tuscan metropolis. For twenty-one days those victorious microbes had brooded in silence in his poisoned arteries. At the end of that time, they swarmed and declared themselves.[29]

Grant Allen's description of the "victorious microbes" is evocative and moving; it bespeaks an epidemiological narrative closer to the *The Hot Zone* of 1994 than a *fin-de-siècle* novel from 1895. His pinpointing of water is not only accurate according to contemporary scientific discourse of the day, but it also highlights the inevitability of connection through the imagery of flowing water that encircles and undergirds all landmasses. Perhaps more visceral, so to speak, is that the imagery he evokes of water contaminated with fecal matter, as Victorians knew to be the case when typhoid struck, again speaks to the inevitability of our human connection, however uncomfortable that fact may be. "It may seem too disgusting for belief," one contemporary article on typhoid explains, "but it is none the less true, that we receive these diseases by inhaling from the air we breathe, or swallowing in the water we drink, particles of *fæcal matter*."[30] Additionally, while Herminia's death emphasizes the failure of any and all isolationist endeavors, Alan's death of typhoid hints at possible successful modes of resistance. The inclusion of typhoid signals innovative contemporary waste disposal methodologies, which emphasized connectivity, openness to risk, and the vitalizing connections with the others who might be abjectified and deemed impure.

Sewage, Flow, and Openness to Risk in Late-Century Typhoid Discourse

This late period of the century was the so-called heyday of microbe hunting—the popular zeal for germ theory. In this time, particularly after the CDA had been repealed and it was an increasingly recognized reality that disease does not obey gender or class boundaries, Victorian science saw a slow but steady rhetorical shift away from isolationist ideology. Periodicals in this era bear witness to the early incorporation of language and practices that speak to the impossibilities of maintaining purity in hermetically sealed vacuums of isolation. Instead, scientific discourse of the very last parts of the century slowly began to promote the same ideas that authors of anti-isolationist literature had been advocating for decades. That is, such perfectly quarantined moral and biological antisepsis was not possible and, even if it were, would backfire and disease the whole of society instead of protecting the purity of isolated individuals. Typhoid in particular illustrated—perhaps more than any other disease—the unsustainability of sequestering the "unclean." After the sanitation movement of the 1840s and 1850s, human waste was typically dumped in closed, underground sewers that led to nearby rivers, the idea being to get as much distance between communities and unwanted waste as quickly as possible. An 1867 handbook on sewage disposal summarizes this history quite well:

> At th[e] [early] period in the history of sanitary reform, the pioneers of science were so impressed with the enormity of the evils arising from retaining decomposing matter in the vicinity of our dwellings, that they were led to look upon sewage as a nuisance to be got rid of as quickly as possible; so they poured it into the nearest stream or watercourse, in the hope that the stream would bear it harmlessly to the ocean, where it would be entombed for ever from sight; but the result has proved different from what we expected. Nature rebels against the waste.[31]

As historian Christopher Hamlin explains, this method involved "simply pouring sewage into a large body of water and hoping for the best."[32] Such plans for sewage disposal (sequestering it and then shuttling it out of sight and far away via waterways) obviously built upon the ideologies of germ theory, which implicitly promoted the desirability of hermetically sealing off, containing, and removing exposure to impurities. However, late-century research into sewage and fecal-oral diseases began to demonstrate that semi-open, aerated systems and *probiotic* development were the only sustainable means of handling the millions of tons of human waste produced daily in England. In addition to the concerns listed above with hoping human waste would simply disappear in waterways, the closed-sewer system was also despaired of. One discussion on the topic explains the dangers of enclosed, sealed refuse: "the great evil to be guarded against . . . with either water or sewage, is stagnation."[33] Another late-century treatise affirms the value of probiotics, explaining that such beneficial microbes, which are "the chief agents in setting up fermentative . . . changes," fail to grow in closed vacuums, and adding that "if sewage be placed in hermetically sealed flasks and sterilized by heat it will be found that these changes do not occur."[34] Instead, a festering build-up and overflow would occur.

These conceptual changes also brought about shifting visual perceptions of microbiological life. As early as the late 1850s, scientists began to take a rather appreciative stance:

> Collective specimens of this suspended organic matter may be found in the quieter parts floating on the surface [of the water]. When submitted to the microscope this . . . substance presents an exceedingly interesting appearance. In it we have collected . . . the graceful and varied forms of several species of animal and vegetable infusoriæ. On closer examination it is soon perceived that these minute creatures are busily engaged in the work of assimilating . . . the softer parts of decayed vegetation into their own organism. In a word, what oxygen does for extractive matter, it is clear that these infinitesimal creatures are performing.[35]

Here, instead of a revolting fear of germs or disgust at their presence, they are anthropomorphized as "busy," effective workers in an environmental factory, "graceful[ly]" processing components of waste, so that they are not left to fester. Instead of bogeymen, readers are presented with servicemen who exist in wondrous and vital symbiosis to humans, rather than being cast as undifferentiated, threatening "others." In fact, a great deal of scientific and engineering literature on the topic at this time not only promotes the value of probiotic breakdown of human refuse and waste but also highlights its utility as fertilizer. Suddenly bacteria were no longer universally to be feared but were instead cast as essential in preventing overflow of waste, while also being helpful in replenishing agricultural environments depleted by humans. One long treatise, *Bacterial Treatment of Sewage*, explains this cyclical process:

> Now just as soil contains these Economic Organisms whose *role* is to complete the cycle of nature, removing the dead remains of plants and animals and assimilating them in such a way as to add to the fertility of the soil and recommence the cycle of life, so also in sewage we have *all the required organisms normally present*, whose business it is to render soluble the solid matters, and to split up the organic compounds into their simple elements,

and then as a final stage in the process to oxidise these elements and so produce and effluent free from putrescible matter, but containing nitrates and other mineral substances.[36]

Significantly, the agricultural environment itself is generally posited as the best means of purifying the sewage, providing the best environment for bacteria to do such work. This mutually constitutive cycle of earth-as-fodder for bacterial purification of waste, and purifying bacteria as food for the same soil, notably functions *outside* of the Anthropocene. Of course, treatises at the time looked for ways to harness these capabilities with the help of human engineering, but their terminology about the benefits of bacteria represent quite a discursive shift from earlier decades in the century. In fact, aversion to such microbiological processes (often represented by the sanitary-era water closet in these engineering tracts) is disavowed as wrongheaded and unethical for its sheer wastefulness grounded in nothing but self-interest—as *Bacterial Treatment of Sewage* explains, the presence of bacteria in sewage "even in very large numbers, is not matter for regret but far otherwise."[37] There was indeed a vocal movement against water closet disposal of sewage, based somewhat on the popularity of "land treatment" of sewage. In *Sewage Purification Brought Up to Date, 1896*, the author, E. Bailey-Denton, acknowledges that "no one familiar with the subject" could "den[y] that the most effective treatment of sewage was . . . passing it through land."[38] Although several methods of probiotic sewage disposal were used, most involved passing sewage through several layers of filtering material of "flint, coke, and gravel," and then passed through to "fine grain bacteria beds" called "cultivation beds" or "contact beds."[39] For the first time, bacteria are applauded and promoted—"cultivated" as any other agricultural life form—not inside a sealed, sanitized laboratory, but in the world of people, animals, and crops.

Generally this probiotic irrigation and fertilization still involved piping the sewage in and, of course, using some amount of water as a vehicle. However, the proven abilities of land itself to purify sewage and sewage to fertilize land, respectively, brought about notions of the "dry closet" as a possibility even superior to the water closet. Earth closets, as they were also called, were essentially indoor outhouses using only dry earth to cover human waste, and this retrograde movement toward approving an entirely open cesspit demonstrates the rhetorical heft that the probiotic movement gained in this last decade of the century. Obviously, the water closet has prevailed, but nevertheless, waste piped to agricultural regions as a fertilizer continued for some time, and the very advocacy surrounding the earth closet at this time is testament to the new fervor about openness, aeration, and connectivity. "Of all our domestic institutions," one sewage handbook claims,

> the water closet system is the most extravagant, the most wasteful, and the most dangerous to human life. The W.C. system found in the houses of the upper ten thousand is the most filthy and hateful, and those as old as the hills, must soon disappear from every household.[40]

Thus, in the late century, scientific and engineering discourse on human waste inverted previously predominant rhetoric: the bacteria are busy, effective workers, ideologically aligned with the middle class, and the "upper ten thousand" are wasteful and promulgate disease with their unwillingness to see their own complicity in it. Instead, openness and connection are emphasized as inevitable and healthy. As one treatise for the dry closet, written by famed sewage engineer G. V. Poore expounds, "the principle is . . . thorough exposure to the air, and if the sunlight have access also so much the better."[41] Another advocate of the dry closet system of probiotics opens his handbook with the provocative statement, "Well may the Chinese call *us* barbarians; in that strange and curious country, containing, according to some authorities, 500 millions of people, such a thing as a W.C. is not to be found."[42] He continues:

> In these days blood poisoning is very common, and in most instances may be traced to the pernicious gases generated in the sewers of towns, to which every W.C. largely contributes. It is only a very few years since the health of our future king was seriously jeopardized by the sewer gas arising from the W.C. at Sandringham. Fortunately, the Prince survived the attack, and this fact will do much to draw the attention of medical men and sanitary authorities to the dangers attending the hateful and filthy plan.[43]

As this passage makes clear, in the later parts of the century, typhoid was the most-publicized consequence of improper waste disposal, particularly after Prince Edward VII came down with a severe bout of typhoid in 1871. His illness and recovery were widely discussed in periodicals of the time, illustrating in high relief the invisible connections among all humans—rich and poor, aristocrat and pauper—that disease forces us to confront. Of course, his father before him famously died of typhoid, something no Victorian reader was liable to forget. One handbook on typhoid titled *Typhoid and Other Allied Diseases* (1876) opens with a reminder of these facts, noting that diseases of "excremental filth" are "as common among the rich as among the poor; the prince may fall their victim as readily as may the peasant, for their horrible cause penetrates to the mansion or the palace as easily as it enters the cottage."[44]

Increasingly, studies showed that bacteria themselves were the best solution for breaking down infectious matter in sewage and, moreover, that the kind of bacteria best at doing this needed airflow and contact with the outside environment to do their job well. Whether dry or wet closets were advocated by a given author, ventilation was always agreed upon as most important—not simply distancing from the refuse or sealing it up. In *How to Make a House Sanitary*, the section on water closets insists that "there should be a ventilating tube through the roof," adding that "windows should be open" in addition, and the closet should never be sequestered "in the basement."[45] The same handbook, in the following sections on privies, cesspools, and the pail system, always notes "it should be ventilated," describing the general rule that pipes as a whole "should act as ventilators."[46] G. V. Poore, in his discussion of earth closets, similarly notes the importance of "cross-ventilation."[47] Closed pipes were liable only to corrosion, and "ventilated soil-pipes resist . . . this corrosive action for a longer period than non-ventilated."[48] In general, most sewage handbooks agreed that periodically placed ventilating devices on pipes were the best method, and such devices are often still used today (see Figure 5.1).[49]

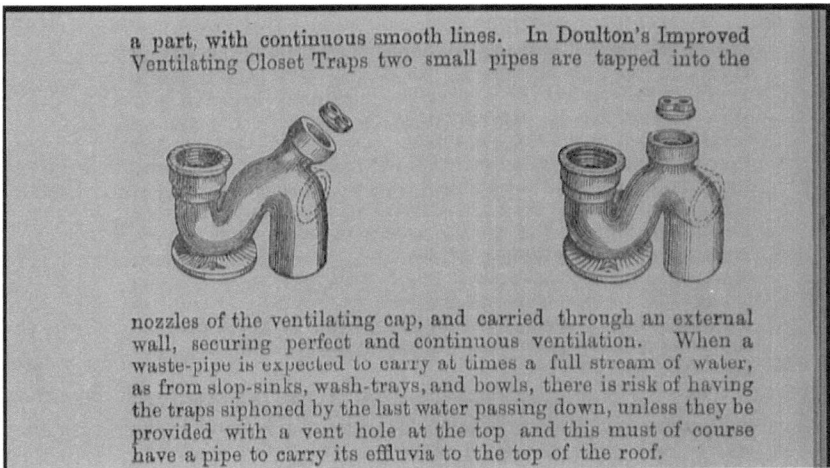

Figure 5.1. Image of Plumbing Ventilation Model, 1877.

Although, as Michelle Allen notes, "by opening a channel of com-munication between the 'outer air' and the interior chamber . . . the sewer posed a threat to the ideals of privacy and autonomy cultivated in and represented by the home," by this point in the century scientific dis-course was aligning itself with the literary endeavors covered in this book in insisting that such was not only inevitable, but necessary.[50] The sewer connected all people and was "an aggressively unifying force."[51] But as the Golden Era of microbe hunting reached its twilight, the prevailing bioethical admonition seemed to be to accept that this unity had always existed in other forms and was, as the previously quoted sewer engineer put it, "not matter for regret, but far otherwise."[52] This notion of planned, mitigated exposures echoes Defoe's much earlier. These findings served, perhaps more than any studies since vaccination experiments and debates, to circulate and promote the idea that bacteria are a risk that must be confronted and even facilitated for *healthy* human life to thrive. Such findings about the actual biological safety net provided by seemingly dangerous microbiological organisms had vast ideological import for humans and their post-germ-theory impulses to isolate themselves from risky and dangerous "other" human bodies. The reviled abject was now publicly discussed as a necessary part of the subject's continued livelihood. That is, much as Defoe insisted so many years earlier, controlled risk exposures are indeed necessary for the maintenance of biological life. Authors such as Allen, Ibsen, and Hardy incorporated such findings into their work metaphorically in their contin-ued and ever-developing insistence that social risk aversion is devitalizing (as did Defoe, Shelly, James, Wood, and Braddon before them). Others insisted that attempting to maintain personal purity via isolation from such perceived risks simply eats communities away from the inside out and further diseases them, morally and biologically (those authors covered here include Hardy, Ibsen, and Dixon).

In *The Woman Who Did*, these issues of sequestration and purity are explicitly rendered in terms of morality and social decorum, thereby extrapolating the concerns of the previous chapter. That is, in *Ghosts* and *The Woodlanders* and *Jude the Obscure*, disease is laid as a palimpsest over the characters who have tried to maintain a socially acceptable form of pro-priety, communicating much about the futility of their aims and even the poisonous nature of such agendas. In *The Woman Who Did*, Allen pushes this metonymic principle even farther, simply referring to unwanted mores as contagions themselves, and demonstrating the natural human tendency to view all others as contaminating. His tragic story illustrates the damning nature of such beliefs, even when they serve the aims of resistance to the status quo. The protagonist's loss of her partner to typhoid indicates further this insistence on community connections, but aside from this brief episode, contagion and contamination are represented as figurative in the story. In Ibsen's 1883 *An Enemy of the People*, the pendulum swings precisely to the opposite polarity, in that the presence of real, physical disease (the potential threat of typhoid fever, to be exact) is the central action that moves the plot, and the implications for human morality in isolation act as rather a subtext to this drama and are easy to miss. In fact, I will present a revisionist reading and argue that far too many scholars *have* missed this important subtext and misread the play entirely.

Finding "The Folk's Fiend" in Ibsen's *En Folkefiende*

The plot of *An Enemy of the People* is deceptively simple. An 1895 *New York Times* review praised Ibsen's "superior constructive skill and facility as a writer of stage dialogue," but wryly noted that "the interest aroused" by the plot was "never very deep or absorbing."[53] A year earlier, the London-based *Referee* claimed that the plot was simply too boring to "command the sympathy of an audience."[54] In fact, up to the present day, the play "has been considered by many Ibsen supporters to be one of the thematically most underdeveloped and baldly didactic of his plays."[55] Thomas F. Van Laan puts the matter more gently, describing it as one of Ibsen's "most straightforward plays ever, lacking almost entirely the hallmarks of complexity and ambiguity" so typical of his work.[56] Indeed, in her 2006 Key Note Presentation at the International Ibsen conference, Merete Morken Andersen opens by acknowledging that

> it is as if the characters are not real characters, not the way we are used to them in Ibsen's plays; they seem to be more of a type cast. Certainly they are more so than the characters in *Ghosts*. . . . We do not get to know much about the inner life of the characters, and there is not much nuance in the way they act.[57]

The plot is simply summarized: in a town where the economy depends upon tourists visiting the local therapeutic baths and spas, the newly hired Dr. Stockmann has discovered bacteria in the water, which he believes are linked to some previously observed cases of typhoid fever. Stockmann announces his findings to the town authorities—a set of local journalists and political figures—along with his recommendation that the baths must be closed indefinitely. When he does so, he is convinced he will be regaled as a local hero. He is shocked when he is met with anger and disbelief for his findings. Later, he calls a town meeting to announce his findings to the public, and again, is deemed no hero, but rather run out of town by a mob shouting "En folkefiende! En folkefiende!" after him as he flees. Although the majority of the town may indeed deem him "an enemy of the people," Dr. Stockmann closes the play seemingly unperturbed, concluding that "the strongest man in the world is the man who stands alone."[58]

It should come as no surprise that I will be arguing against the viability of Stockmann's closing assertion. But before explicating my longer arguments and interpretations about the play, it is worth taking a moment to review how Stockmann has traditionally been read: as a morally upright, sole exemplar of ecocritical truths, the sole bastion of morality in a sea of depravity. Interpretations of the play have cast Dr. Stockmann as a hero of the people, and his epithet of "an enemy of the people" as uncomplicated evidence of the corruption of the society around him. The title alone of one 2003 article on the topic, "*Dr. Stockmann og Dr. Snow—to samfunnsmedisinske helter*" (Dr. Stockmann and Dr. Snow—two social medicine heroes) is quite representative of this traditional reading.[59] This article critiques some aspects of Stockmann's approach, but ultimately concludes that he is "*velmmenende, men naiv*" (well-meaning but naive).[60] A response article written in support of this one casts Stockmann as "a symbolic beacon in the night for modern public health activists."[61] A 2008 article describes Stockmann as a victim of "greed and ignorance," who is "battered by the gales of ignorance and prejudice," ultimately labeling Stockmann a "truth-teller."[62] A thorough literature review of Stockmann's interpretation can be found in Thomas F. Van Laan's 1986 article on the play, but his summation is worth quoting here: "From its appearance," he notes, "commentators have been inclined to adhere to a single uncomplicated reading of the play" as a simple depiction of a "protagonist's struggles against a mob of 'crooks and fools' and his ultimate spiritual triumph in the midst of practical and material defeat."[63]

Such readings fail to take into account, however, Stockmann's biopolitical ideologies represented in both his scientific methodologies and the nature of his town hall speech that directly precedes his forced exile. These elements will compose the bulk of my own interpretation of the play. First of all,

Stockmann perfectly espouses the isolationist imperatives of germ theory's insistence on quarantine and purity when he insists that the entire town must shut down because of his isolated belief that the water is dangerous. This becomes even clearer during his town hall speech, in which he proclaims that he alone can access epistemological truths and should rule society as an autocrat. Thus, the public outcry against him can itself be seen as the broad embodiment of the aims of the literature covered in the previous chapters. That is, by labeling Stockmann a "*folkefiende*"—a fiend of the folk, or, as it has most frequently been translated, "an enemy of the people"—the townsfolk are in fact labeling bacteriology's ideology as the enemy of the people rather than its savior. The authors I have covered in this book all speak out against self-interested moral and biological isolation, a stance they conclude ignores community needs and connection. As the embodiment of this movement, the townsfolk in *An Enemy of the People* cry foul of germ theory's fallout. If this were not clear enough from the basic plot, Stockmann's own speech to the town makes this, I would argue, abundantly clear. When he meets with the townspeople, ostensibly to persuade them of the need for the closure of the town, instead of speaking of his own scientific findings, he spends his entire stage time asserting the moral rectitude of leadership by an intellectual elite who simply "know better" than the majority. He opens by suddenly announcing that he has "more important things to speak about" than "this petty business about the water-supply being polluted and the Baths standing over a cesspool."[64] Instead, he tells the townspeople, he is going to discuss the manner in which "our *spiritual* sources are polluted and that our whole civic community is built over a cesspool of lies."[65] Thus far, it would seem that *An Enemy of the People* simply reconfigures the concerns of *Ghosts*. Stockmann's unsavory motivations are quickly apparent, however. Rather than discussing his disgust with the opposition he faces from the mayor and local media (whose motivations are uncertain), he quickly moves on to proclaiming that he, and intellectuals like him, should control society. "The worst enemy of truth and freedom in our society," he continues, is "the damned, compact, liberal majority."[66] Coming on the heels of *Ghosts*, this proclamation could well seem to be simply another condemnation of the moral status quo and middle-class propriety. But Stockmann is far from finished. His speech continues:

> The majority is never right. Never, I tell you. . . . Who are the people that make up the biggest proportion of the population—

the intelligent ones or the fools? I think we can agree it's the
fools, no matter where you go in this world it's the fools that
form the overwhelming majority. But I'll be damned if that means
it's right that the fools should dominate the intelligent. . . . The
majority has the *might*—more's the pity—but it hasn't *right*.[67]

So far, Stockmann does not appear in an entirely reprehensible light. But
he keeps talking. "*I* am right," he declares, "I and one or two other individuals like me. The minority is always right."[68] While he reproduces the
society-as-diseased rhetoric seen in *Ghosts*, the more he speaks (and his
diatribe continues for pages), the more dissonant his rhetorical parallels
become. He claims that "this damned compact majority—*this* is the thing
that's polluting the sources of our spiritual life and infecting the very ground
we stand on."[69] He calls "majority truths" a "moral scurvy," which seems
rather in line with the messages presented in the previous chapter, that social
norms are themselves diseasing society.[70] However, what critics have failed
to give adequate weight to are the logical conclusions Stockmann draws
from these presumptions. Like Allen, Ibsen presents here a character who
has possibly pinpointed a disease, but has grossly misjudged the remedy in
presenting himself as the sole savior of a society and the single source of
progress and change. As Stockmann continues, his proposed solution (rule
by the intellectual elite) becomes increasingly disturbing:

> [It is] a rotten lie [that] . . . the common herd, the masses are
> the very essence of the people—that they *are* the people—that
> the common man, and all the ignorant and immature elements
> in society have the same right to criticize and to approve, to
> govern and to counsel as the intellectually distinguished people.[71]

It is possible, when selectively choosing his statements, to read Stockmann
as simply arguing against the status quo, as seen in chapter 4. However, as
his arguments develop, his shocking statements that only "the intellectually
distinguished" have "the . . . right to criticize and to approve" the goings-on
in the world around them cannot be taken lightly. He is not simply saying
that there are serious problems with the moral status quo, but that majority
is *always* in the wrong (thus speaking out quite distinctly against democracy
and enfranchisement of the poor), while he "and a few others like" him are
the *only* people *ever* to be trusted with power and authority. Considering,

moreover, that he has called this meeting with the common people of the town, he is in fact speaking to those who are already disempowered and marginalized. This is decidedly so, since Norway was quite a poor country in the nineteenth century, particularly in the rural areas such as the "miserable hole of a . . . rocky wilderness" full of "poor half-starved creatures" where *An Enemy of the People* is explicitly set.[72] His elitism takes on eugenicist tones as he draws an elaborate metaphor between himself as a purebred dog and everyone else as mutts—he has in fact preemptively opened his speech by claiming the populace would be better treated by a "vet" than by a doctor like himself.[73] This passage is worth quoting at length:

> Look at the difference between pedigree and cross-bred animals. . . . Think first of an ordinary mongrel—I mean one of those filthy, shaggy rough dogs that do nothing but run about the streets and cock their legs against all the walls. Compare a mongrel like that with a poodle whose pedigree goes back many generations, who has been properly fed and has grown up among quiet voices and soft music. Don't you think the poodle's brain will have developed quite differently from the mongrel's? You bet it will! That kind of pedigree dog can be trained to do the most fantastic tricks—things an ordinary mongrel could never learn even if it stood on its head.[74]

He continues to insist upon rule by the elite, reiterating that "there's a tremendous difference between the poodles and the mongrels amongst us men."[75] He then turns positively Kurtzian, arguing for the extermination of all the masses:

> When a place has become riddled with lies, who cares if it's destroyed? I say it should simply be razed to the ground! And all the people living by these lies should be wiped out, like vermin! You'll have the whole country infested in the end, so that eventually the whole country deserves to be destroyed.[76]

He maintains his belief in his own individual moral superiority to the end of the play. Even after he is run out of town, Stockmann's most horrific memory of the violent mob is "the idea of the mob going for me as though they were my equals—*that's* what I can't stomach, damn it!"[77]

Remarkably, nearly every critical writing on Stockmann, including modern-day performances of the plays and adaptations of it, neatly sidestep his quasi-fascist arguments. Arthur Miller famously redacted this entire speech when writing a modern adaptation of the play, citing "discomfort" with his support of "an evolving aristocracy of leaders with broad powers to mould community standards."[78] At most, some sources describe him as naive or bad at public communication of scientific findings to lay people (a view, which, to my thinking, tends to reify Stockmann's own disdain for lay persons).[79] Paul Lindholdt at least acknowledges "the troubling strain in Stockmann's speech," but chalks it up to "the rudimentary state of anthropology and the social science at the time."[80] Such excuses for Stockmann fall flat, however, in light of the support for increasing enfranchisement in the late periods of the century.

This rendering of the bacteriological biopolitical agenda is nearly farcical as Stockmann proclaims, on the basis of his visual perception of germs in the town water, that he and a select few men of science like him have the right to authoritarian rule. Such claims are astounding. Perhaps it is even more astounding that these claims have been comfortably elided by interpreters of this play, who continue to uphold Stockmann as an innocent victim of an evil society, a besieged whistleblower who attempts to do good and save his town. In fact, although he has almost never been seriously viewed as an enemy of the people (as I argue that he in fact is), contemporary Victorian critics and audiences seemed at least a great deal more willing to acknowledge Stockmann's fascist agenda. I will argue momentarily that this is because they were more connected to the scientific processes of their own day; our own myopia of these methodologies allows us to simply take his initial empirical observations at face value, and enable easy, uncritical acceptance of his ultimate conclusions. Many reviews did uphold the view of Stockmann as a hero; however, there seems to have been less unanimity in this view in the nineteenth century than today. I have earlier called his reasoning (from disease germ to dictatorship) farcical; the Victorians tended to cast its extremism as satirical. "He leaps to some startling convictions," a 1909 review concludes, "concerning majorities and democracy."[81] This same review remarks that he "comes off at last the moral victor," however, but goes farther toward at least acknowledging Stockmann's dictatorial ethos than present-day criticism.[82] The play, it concludes, "may be classed as a straightforward satiric comedy."[83] A much earlier review, from 1893, recounts that "the piece was received with the wildest enthusiasm" by the audience, even in spite of the fact that "the hero of it, *as is well known,* does not believe in democracy."[84] In 1893, then, ten years after the play's first premiere, it was "well known" to nineteenth-century audiences that Stockmann was antidemocratic, at best. A review a year later dubbed the play, as many were wont to do, "a lumpish satire" in which "Stockmann simply insults the meeting that had been called for a very different purpose."[85] One reviewer utterly throws his hands up, exclaiming that

> nobody can pretend to analyze [Ibsen] for the very simple reason that hardly any two people think alike about him. In this case, for instance, he may have meant to indict the "compact majority" and to establish the corollary of the man who stands alone. On the other hand, he may have intended to exploit the irrationality of extreme theory in practice.[86]

In his native Norway, *An Enemy of the People* was one of the first plays produced during the first season of Norway's National Theater.[87] The theater was built upon lofty principles of liberty and free speech, anticipated eloquently during its construction:

> *Nationaltheatret har af den norske stat intent tilskud; det nyder af staten ingen rettigheder—men har derfor på anden side ligeoverfor staten heller ingen forpligtelser.*

> The National Theater receives no subsidies from the state. Thus, while it has no rights accorded to it from the state, on the other hand, it has no obligations to the state, either.[88]

It is certainly hard to imagine that this play would have been carefully selected for the first season of a theater with incredibly liberal principles if contemporary Norwegians saw the play as espousing aristocratic, dictatorial reign.

Somewhere along the way, however, literary critics have lost the ability or willingness to take Stockmann at his word, and have chosen to either excuse or ignore his totalitarian philosophy that was readily apparent to contemporary audiences. Instead, as a promotional poster from 1991 dramatically entices, he is cast and recast as a character who "is fighting to reveal the truth—and save people's lives" (see Figure 5.2).

Yet in his own words, Stockmann doesn't seem to think people are worth saving. Indeed, a careful review of his discovery of the germs in the water reveals not his shock and horror at the dangers revealed, but rather excitement that he will finally make his name as a famous scientist. Throughout the play, Stockmann is consistent in his excitement that what are apparently dangerous findings will bring him renown; he is much less concerned about the supposed danger people may or may not be in. From the first, he describes what should be distressing findings as "a great discovery."[89] As he explains his findings with his wife, he talks with excitement about his hopes for an improvement in his reputation:

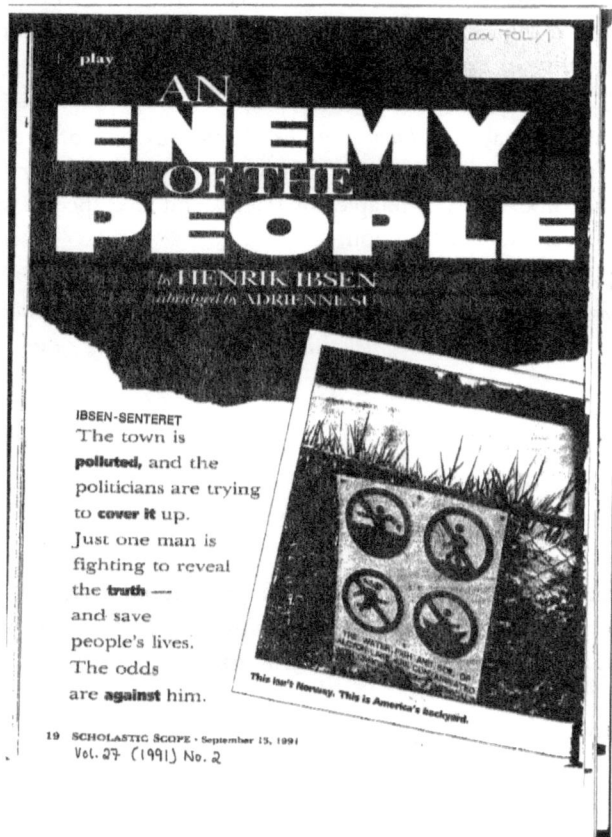

Figure 5.2. Press Release for An Enemy of the People Production, 1991.

DR. STOCKMANN: All right, to your grandfather, then. Yes, now we'll give that old boy something that will really open his eyes. He's another one that thinks I'm a bit cracked—oh yes, there are plenty more with the same idea, I can see. But now these good people are going to see something—they're certainly going to see something, this time. [*He walks around rubbing his hands.*] What a commotion this is going to cause in town, Katherine! You've no idea! All the pipes will have to be relaid.

In this excerpt, Stockmann is oddly excited about a discovery that, if true, will mean financial disaster for all of his neighbors (we are told that the remedies he suggests will cost "several hundred thousand crowns" and that he demands the entire town be closed down while funds are raised and improvements made).[90] Well may the Victorians have called the play a satire, as Stockmann imagines the downfall of the town while rubbing his hands together like a villain from a melodrama. His tone is rather like a gossipmonger as he envisions "the commotion" his scientific analyses will cause in town, and he then returns to the mode of melodramatic villain as he imagines the Baths as the " 'artery' of the town," its "throbbing heart," and simultaneously imagines himself stopping its pulsing flow.[91] Circulatory imagery has been used by many authors covered in this book, and it is apt here as well. Stagnation is ubiquitously used by these authors to indicate the poisonous putrefaction brought about by isolationist impulses. Here, Stockmann's moral isolation, like Herminia's, is the cause of his downfall, and he is cast in the first scene of the play as not only a proponent of stagnation, of isolation and "purity," but also as an actual murderer, fantasizing about stopping a heartbeat. Of course, as the play later reveals, he actually disavows the innate value of the hearts, minds, and bodies of his fellow citizens. He deems them ill-bred dogs with no right to free will and demands their extermination. Certainly the "beating heart" of their community and its financial stability are expendable to him, as well. His joy at discovering something potentially so tragic and his immediate conclusions that such findings render him a fit dictator of an entire society are, I would argue, unavoidably problematic. Is it really any surprise that the townspeople run him out of town, calling him a public enemy? Especially in light of the current Western political climate, it seems hard to argue with the townspeople's motivations. Although Stockmann does not publicly proclaim his unique capabilities as a dictator until the play's conclusion, he excitedly imagines the ruin he will bring to the town and

his concomitant rise as a "man of science" (as he repeatedly calls himself)
brought about by his discoveries.[92]

Recall that this is the height of the figure Paul DeKruif called "the
microbe hunter," a scientist-hero tirelessly venturing forth to shed light on
the foul effluvia infecting society. Pasteur had already gained great fame in
this manner, as had John Snow before him (and before germ theory itself).
Koch bootstrapped his way to fame and fortune from humble beginnings
by entering the microbe-hunting trade.[93] Stockmann clearly aspires more to
personal glory than to public safety. Moreover, one could even argue that
Stockmann is so eager to gain fame as a microbe hunter that he jumps the
gun, so to speak, employing questionable scientific methodologies according
to contemporary scientific standards—something not lost on Victorian audiences. For one, he does not even perform his own microbe-hunting work.
As a self-proclaimed "man of science," he admits that he does not have "the
necessary scientific equipment" to study the town water adequately himself.[94]
Instead, he sends the water off to a lab for "exact chemical analysis," and
then tries to take credit for others' microbe-hunting work.[95] Moreover, "his"
findings are not necessarily replicable, a notion important to the scientific
method even at this time.[96] The idea that the entire town must be shut
down immediately based on one single water sample, analyzed by one single
lab whose findings are provided secondhand, is dubious. At the very least,
it seems that the people of the town are more reasonable than otherwise to
question just how "scrupulous[ly] thorough" (as he terms it) his investigations
were, rather than accepting them as a matter of course.

Finally, his epidemiological reasoning is unsound to begin with.
Stockmann claims that he began to have "suspicions" about the water after
a "number of curious cases of sickness among the visitors . . . typhoid and
gastric fever . . ." the previous winter.[97] His suspicions caused him to send
the water for analysis. After bacteria are found in the water, he claims his
suspicions are confirmed and the entire industry of the town must be shut
down. Koch's principles, well established at this point, required that to assume
a given microbe was causing a disease, it had to be: (1) isolated from an
ill organism; (2) cultured in a Petri dish; (3) extracted from said media;
(4) inoculated into another living organism; and (5) observed to cause the
same disease in the second individual. Stockmann has not only not gone
through this process, he has outsourced the few observations he has made,
and he has made a huge assumptive leap by causally joining his empirical
observation of illness and separate, independent observation of "organisms"
(not necessarily typhoid bacteria) in water. From these unlinked observations, he sees fit to claim both authority as a microbe hunter via praxis

(which he in fact outsources) and epidemiological reasoning (which he has completely forgone). Instead of a linked chain of epidemiological evidence, Stockmann makes two discrete observations and links them causally in lieu of any further evidence suggesting the veracity of doing so.

Moreover, as mentioned earlier, contemporary studies of sewage and waste disposal found that in fact many bacteria were incredibly helpful, and many discussions of sewage from this period go to great lengths to convince readers that bacteria in water did not necessarily indicate the presence of disease. For one, most bacteria had been found by this time to be either innocuous or beneficial. Secondly, scientists argued that Darwinian principles of competition caused even the presence of harmful bacteria to be rather inept due to crowding and resource competition in properly ventilated, willingly cultivated sewer biomes. *The Bacteriology of Sewage* explains that, given

> such a large quantity of organic matter as sewage contains . . . there is but one reason why such a medium is not absolutely ideal from a microbe's point of view, and that reason is that in sewage the vast numbers of bacteria present make the struggle for existence exceptionally keen.[98]

The explanation continues: "Not only are the numbers incredibly large, but we also find an extensive representation of species, including . . . non-pathogenic and pathogenic."[99] After describing some common varietals, the author concludes by urging his readers not to be overly concerned about typhoid in sewage: "In crude unsterilized sewage it is clear that owing to competition and the inimical effect some of the non-pathogenic species have upon *B. typhosus,* that the death of that organism in sewage" is likely.[100] Thus, not only are Stockmann's reasoning faulty and methodology flawed, but his findings have the potential to dangerously backfire. Probiotic sources tend to break down *B. typhosus,* so without following any sort of protocol, Stockmann risks instead "cleansing" beneficial bacteria, thus disrupting the microbiome and allowing for an overgrowth and outbreak of the very bacteria he claims to be concerned about. Once again, we see here a text in which attempts at maintaining a perfect form of purity are ticking time bombs causing stagnation, putrefaction, and overflow. The attempted remedy causes the disease once more, as the authors covered in this book have repeatedly demonstrated.

Indeed, contemporary reviews wondered at his claims. One Danish review from 1883 describes his findings as *"altfor trivielle"* ("overly trivial.")[101] Moreover, the review adds,

Næsten alt hvad han siget i sin store Tale er enten meningløst eller selvindlysende, de var unødvendigt at tromme saamange Mennesker sammen for at høre det.

Nearly everything he says in his lengthy speech is either so meaningless or obvious, that it was unnecessary to assemble together so many people to hear it.[102]

Thus, while Stockmann presents himself as a "man of science" who does "scientific tests," he is not doing his own work, he is not doing the right kind of work, and he is not doing it in the right order. And yet critics have typically interpreted him, nevertheless, as a sort of example of moral fortitude. I would suggest that if he is an example of any kind of moral fortitude, it is only that of upholding the status quo of germ theory biopolitical implications (although not necessarily what microbiologists themselves would have consciously intended), which suggests humans *can* exist and thrive in a vacuum, while disregarding the rest of society (as his closing lines indeed indicate). Instead, when read through the lens of other works of literature resisting the biopolitical admonitions of the age, Stockmann is a straw man, promoting the moral and physical quarantine that contemporary authors and contemporary engineers revealed as explosive.

One other possibility needs to be addressed. While most critics of the play either completely ignore Stockmann's problematic fascist biopolitics based on problematic scientific reasoning, some have read Stockmann as an obvious stand-in for Ibsen himself and therefore intended by Ibsen to be viewed positively. Ibsen did write *An Enemy of the People* directly after his social critiques in *Ghosts* situated him at the epicenter of public disapproval. Thus, many read Stockmann as Ibsen's own self-portrait, of a valiant hero trying to shed light on a corrupt society who castigates the hero for said whistleblowing. Arthur Miller called this idea—that "Ibsen wrote the play as a riposte to those who so violently attacked him as an enemy of society for having written *Ghosts*—"an assumption that [he] never questioned."[103] Many critics posit this idea as plain fact, such as Bernard Dukore, who says, "Dr. Stockmann's interpretation of events is Ibsen's."[104] Paul Lindholdt acknowledges that "consensus rests on a strongly autobiographical basis for Ibsen's composing *An Enemy of the People*."[105] However, Ibsen mocked Stockmann as a character who was "strange," "foolhardy," and "muddleheaded."[106] When asked directly if he agreed with Stockmann's final sentiments in the play, Ibsen quite matter-of-factly argued, "I am not responsible for all the nonsense which

[Dr. Stockmann]" produces.[107] When pressed about the seeming sympathy between himself and his protagonist, he retorted: "Do you really think you know that? Perhaps you are completely wrong," further calling Stockmann "muddle-headed."[108] Thus, as with Grant Allen's *The Woman Who Did* (and as I will argue about Hardy's *The Well-Beloved*), we must give Ibsen his due as an artist capable of producing more than purely autobiographical fantasies. Moreover, as Allen and Ibsen depict such obviously flawed characters who fail at achieving their goals because of these flaws, critics and readers alike would do well to separate the artist from the art. Particularly insofar as contemporary reception of both works picked up so universally on the doomed strategies of these characters, highlighting such as distinct from the artistic prowess of the authors, it seems worthwhile to consider that such authors were capable of representing something outside of their own perspectives and that they depicted fatal flaws and human failings precisely as such, and not necessarily as heavy-handed, martyred autobiographies.

I have mentioned previously the connections between typhoid fever and late-century sewerage developments. Of course, the most famous events involving waste and disease in the Victorian era involved cholera much earlier in the century. It is significant, then, that in *An Enemy of the People*, Ibsen presents typhoid as the feared contagion, not cholera. This is, in fact, a point many critics have used to support the autobiographical nature of the play, as Ibsen apparently based the story on a cholera outbreak in a bathing town.[109] However, I would conversely argue that this proves just the opposite, as Ibsen's update to his source material demonstrates that he elected to work with more prescient concerns of his time. Moreover, it was cholera initially that brought about some of the earlier modes of handling waste (such as casting it into the river or locking it up in a sealed tank) which the later typhoid investigations reversed, emphasizing instead openness and vented systems with mediated exposure, contact, and risk. This open-flow system of handling contaminants and ideologically threatening (if not biologically so) germs functioned as a neat overlay for authors' concerns about human society in a world of risk. In fact, many contemporary critics highlighted Ibsen's play as one showing the failures of such extremism, demonstrated by his insistence on perfect purity and his own moral superiority. The 1883 Danish review proclaimed the falsehood of Stockmann's extremism as statistically impossible. Another review pokes fun at readers who agree with Stockmann and clumsily read him as a hero, arguing that "if the 'compact majority' be a failure so stupendous as some people read it . . . and if the select few know it all, there is obviously no middle course. The only retreat, then, is to absolutism."[110] The aforementioned 1909 review insists that Stockmann's recommendations cannot be taken seriously by the populace or the audience:

> [Ibsen] by no means intends to convey, all the time, that the worthy doctor's [bacteria] actually endangered [the town]. Some of the time, on the contrary—if not a good part of it, he caricatures the doctor himself. Nobody knows better than Ibsen that if some of the worthy doctors had their way we should eat next to nothing and perish for want of water and all for fear of [bacteria].[111]

Thus, when Stockmann insists that the strongest is he who stands alone, Ibsen—by incorporating typhoid into his plot—is alluding to the unviability of isolationist politics via implicit suggestion of the imagery of failed efforts to seal off waste and contaminants that resulted in nothing less than festering and overflow. A successful system mitigates this risk, avoids extremism, and remains open to the outside world, and effectively leans *into* the inextricably connection of one human to the world of other humans around them.

Sewage as a Metaphor for Free Love in Hardy's Final Novel

This brings me to my final text in this chapter, which I will cover only briefly by way of conclusion, Thomas Hardy's odd and oft-reviled (particularly by present-day critics) novel *The Well-Beloved*. I'm concerned here chiefly with Hardy's theoretical and philosophical aims in crafting the nebulous figure of "the well-beloved," and will not cover the intricacies of the plot itself. Written first in 1892 and then rewritten in 1897, both before and after, then, the publication of *Jude the Obscure* in 1895, *The Well-Beloved* is the story of Jocelyn Pierston, an up-and-coming sculptor who lives in the remote Dorset island of Portland. During the novel, he leaves the island and moves to London, joining the Royal Society as a famed artist. This, however, is mere backdrop to the true plot of the story—the movement of Pierston's "well-beloved," a palimpsestic euphemism describing the capriciousness of his own sexual attraction. During the novel, Pierston falls in love with Avice Caro. Then he falls in love with her daughter. Then he falls in love with *her* daughter. Especially given Hardy's own tendencies to become infatuated with women much younger than himself, modern literary scholars tend to react with distaste to the novel. As I have argued with the previous two authors covered in this chapter, however, I would suggest the value of setting aside convenient interpretations of novels as thinly veiled autobiographies. Hardy's own quasi-lecherous tendencies aside, then, this odd pretext of a plot provides, I would argue, a uniquely late-century view of society. In the context of flow and openness, I'd like to highlight the nature of "the well-beloved" as something explicitly tagged as symbolic in the novel. The figure of the well-beloved as a disembodied but living figure is introduced in nearly the first page of the novel as "a migratory, elusive idealization who, ever since his boyhood, had flitted from human shell to human shell." In the 1897 version, Hardy omits the reference to human shells, but maintains his insistence on the disembodied—I would argue symbolic—nature of the well-beloved. His longer explanation of the figure, which follows on the heels of this, remains mostly unchanged between the two versions:

> To his Well-Beloved he had always been faithful; but she had many embodiments. Each individuality known as Lucy, Jane, Flora, Evangeline, or whatnot, had been merely a transient condition of her. He did not recognize this as an excuse or as a defense, but as a fact simply. Essentially she was perhaps of no tangible substance: a spirit, a dream, a frenzy, a conception, an aroma, an epitomized sex, a light of the eye, a parting of the lips. . . . By making this clear to his mind some time before today, he had escaped a good deal of ugly self-reproach [*1897 addition:* which he might otherwise have incurred from his own judgment, as being the very embodiment of fickleness.] It was simply that she who always attracted him, and led him whither she would as by a silken thread, had not remained the occupant of the same fleshly tabernacle in her career so far.[112]

Thus, I would like to suggest in closing that Hardy's use of the well-beloved, as any human entity whose value is suddenly made visible to an observer, was a productive means of highlighting the fact that any human narrative has value, if this value is only attended to. While, indeed, Pierston's own fetishization of women is often difficult to excuse, Hardy in fact makes no excuses for it (as the above passage states rather blatantly). Rather, readers must separate the *character* of Pierston from the narrative voice, and that voice from Hardy's own, all of which are capable of holding different values of the women, both sexual and human. Pierston may make poor use of the well-beloved, that is, but Hardy's figuration of the well-beloved operates by forcing attendance to and focus on the humanity of randomly selected individuals, highlighting through this device (as his work is so wont to do) the value of the small, unnamed experiences of the human, animal, vegetable, and even microbial community around us.

The intensely regional flavor of *The Well-Beloved* also drives this point home. Hardy is well known for highlighting the value of his native Dorset community, all too readily filed away as "backwater" farmers to London readers and other urbanites. More than most Victorian authors, Hardy is always deeply invested with humanizing the Dorset locals and highlighting the value of even those small, little-heard-of communities that may otherwise seem foreign. Thus, readers of Hardy are privy to small-town pub scenes, rural folklore, and folk music from Dorset—all in the name of upholding the value of the small communities which Hardy was privy to. If we can recognize the value of these esoteric practices, surely we can recognize the value of all *people* in the human community.

If Dorset constituted regional fiction about a far-off area to most British Victorians, Portland constitutes its own incredibly isolated area *within* Dorset. Set far off the coast, connected by only a small land-bridge even today, Portland was incredibly insular in the Victorian Era (the land-bridge having yet to be built). Hardy in fact prefaces his 1892 manuscript by highlighting the intensely individual nature of the community in which he sets the story, describing Portland as a "peninsula carved by time out of a single stone, whereon most of the following scenes are laid, has been for centuries immemorial the home of a curious and well-nigh distinct people, cherishing strange beliefs and singular customs."[113] It is significant here that Hardy immediately follows his identification of an isolated place by explaining its relevance to a unique *community* worthy of devoting time and attention to in his novel, in spite of—and Hardy likely would have said because of—their "strange beliefs and singular customs." He continues his preface by anticipating concerns about the unpalatability or uninteresting nature of his depictions, while simultaneously highlighting the symbolic character of the well-beloved itself:

> It is a spot apt to generate a type of personage like the character imperfectly sketched in these pages—a native of natives—whom some may choose to call a fantast (if they honor him with their consideration so far), but whom others may see only as one that gave objective continuity and a name to a delicate dream which

in a vaguer form is more or less common to all men, and is by
no means new to Platonic philosophers.[114]

I have said that Portland is regionalized even within the regionalized Dorset;
Hardy insists that his protagonist is "a native of natives," promoting early
on his narrative call to "honor" others with simple "consideration." The
regionalism and careful attention to humble creatures and characters across
his entire *oeuvre,* and this novel particularly, insists that the vast array of
individualized lives (with which we live in constant communion) warrant
our attention. Moreover, his preface urges, readers would likely find that,
if given, this momentary attention would prove its own worth by raising
awareness of the intrinsic value of this community at large. As I've suggested, for Hardy, this is only possible through intermittent but repeated,
hyper-focused and individualized accounts of experience of the community
and world that provide spaces of empathy and connection through narrative. His emphasis on Platonic forms and types emphasizes his authorial
separation from Pierston, as he introduces the concept of the well-beloved
as something "common to all men" and familiar to Platonists. Pierston's
odd philanderings are by no means "common to all," and his odd fetishes
are certainly portrayed as just that—unique fetishes. Instead, I would argue,
we must take the narrative voice at its word, promoting some element
of Pierston's experiences that can indeed be shared by all, and this is the
promotion throughout the novel of various human types—who represent
simply the form of humanity and its need for connection and empathy as
demonstrated through repeated, episodic, and highlighted focus on them.

The stone upon which the island is formed (mentioned in the first
line of the preface) is also integral to the novel's suggestions about human
community, which I argue draw on sewage developments in the late century.
The landscape of Portland is radically different from the rest of Dorset,
constituted of neither the rolling dairy farms of the Frome Valley, nor the
beautiful sandy beachscapes on the west coast so popular with British tourists
today. The Island of Portland, rather, is imbued with a chalky whiteness that
pervades the atmosphere, and the beaches are comprised of rough shingled
stones. The chalky whiteness is owing to the island's main commodity—
Portland stone—which is hewn all over the island. Portland stone is known
for its unique qualities as a mineral, and was used in late-century sewerage
innovations as a suitably smooth and nonporous material for pipes at this
time. Just as manuals on piping emphasized ventilation, they also emphasized
the import of nonporous surfaces which encouraged flow across them, rather

than absorption and stagnation. In regard to sewer pipes, one handbook urges that "sewers should be made of glazed earthenware, or well-burnt, impervious brick, set in Portland cement."[115] Most handbooks echo this sentiment, emphasizing "enameled," "non-absorbant," or "smooth-glazed surfaces" alongside their emphases on ventilation.[116] The image here emphasizes well the ideological work that such smooth, nonporous pipes did toward insisting on "perfect conductors" of flow (see Figure 5.3).[117]

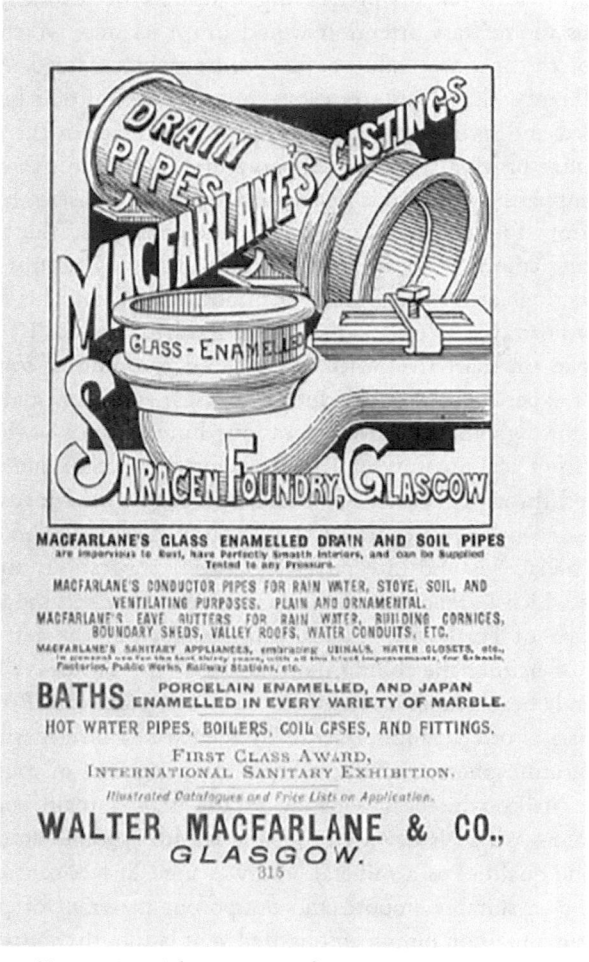

Figure 5.3. Advertisement for Sewage Pipes, 1896.

The figure of the well-beloved can be meaningfully read, I would argue, as an awareness of human value that flits from being to being, alighting for brief periods on individuals as a veritable human interest piece and then moving on, embodying perfectly a flowing conduit highlighting individuals connected through the invisible bonds of community as well as the invisible microbiomes that tie them together. This is especially so, as the novel in the 1892 edition concludes with a reflection on sewage piping. While typhoid is never mentioned in *The Well-Beloved*, the first version of the novel intriguingly concludes with this abrupt embedded epilogue:

> [Pierston's] business was, among kindred undertakings which followed the extinction of the Well-Beloved and other ideals, to advance a scheme for the closing of the old natural fountains in the Street of Wells, because of their possible contamination, and supplying the townlet with water from pipes, a scheme that was carried out at his expense, as is well known. He was also engaged in acquiring some old moss-grown . . . cottages, for the purpose of pulling them down because they were damp; which he afterwards did, and built new ones with hollow walls and full of ventilators.[118]

The once-famous sculptor has ended his career innovating the sewers that rely both on this intensely localized Portland stone and also on flow and ventilation. Once again, we see a human and community setup in a plot that involves the highlighting of human value and connection between humans, overlaid with a palimpsest of the paradoxically relevant discussion of contemporary typhoid and sewerage innovations. Moreover, whereas Pierston's personal fetishized approach to the well-beloved is "extinct," he instead opts for more platonic (double-entendre intended) commitment to the human community that had been symbolically suggested (and subjectively misused by him) throughout the plot. Here, he engages in community improvement projects that primarily highlight the value of flow, connection, and openness to risk (through ventilation). This odd, seemingly irrelevant ending to a novel apparently about very different things brings Hardy's narrative argument about ethical community behavior full circle. Although Pierston may abuse his awareness of the well-beloved throughout the novel, Hardy forces reader attention to the potential benefits of growing awareness of the human community and willingness to engage in and improve it from within, rather than from a place of isolated moral superiority.

In *The Woman Who Did*, readers are privy to the story of a woman's failed attempt to live in moral isolation—disconnected from her fellow man and their plight. Here, typhoid, a disease of festering, sealed sewers, is used to kill off her partner, thus isolating her even beyond her own desires and thereby revealing the problems with attempting to attain purity via isolation. In *An Enemy of the People*, a less-than-scrupulous scientist invokes the specter of this same disease to insist upon his own dictatorial leadership of the populace. Again, the main character's insistence upon isolated moral superiority leads to his downfall, and this tragic ending—in which he insists upon the value of his isolation even as he is attacked by a mob—walks in lockstep with his outdated notions of sealing away physical disease rather than acknowledging the necessary and vital role of connection with risk encounters. Thus, the human and the microbe mutually constitute the moral outcomes of these plots and their implications—nothing is without risk, and risk is in fact vital to humanity's emotional and moral vitality. Finally, in *The Well-Beloved*, Hardy turns the tables entirely—as is so characteristic of his defiant plot stylings—and uses the idea of free love as a paradoxical and provocative means of insisting upon connection and universal human value. This constitutes a shift from Jude and Sue's attempt at progress through moral isolationism, and Hardy closes this book curiously (although I hope it will no longer seem curious) with the only prolonged depiction of cutting-edge sewage disposal that I have personally encountered in Victorian fiction, one that insists upon flow, openness, and connection with the seemingly threatening, all in pursuit of a life more meaningful than mere biological existence. Counterintuitively, then, late-Victorian authors found in representations of human waste a means of urging readers not to waste their ability to see the humanity of others.

Conclusion

Shuffling within Our Mortal Coil

From the contagion of the world's slow stain
He is secure, and now can never mourn
A heart grown cold, a head grown gray in vain;
Nor, when the spirit's self has ceased to burn,
With sparkless ashes load an unlamented urn.

—Percy Shelley, *Adonais*

When I have fears that I may cease to be
Before my pen has gleaned my teeming brain,
Before high‐pilèd books, in charactery,
Hold like rich garners the full ripened grain;
When I behold, upon the night's starred face,
Huge cloudy symbols of a high romance,
And think that I may never live to trace
Their shadows with the magic hand of chance;
And when I feel, fair creature of an hour,
That I shall never look upon thee more,
Never have relish in the faery power
Of unreflecting love—then on the shore
Of the wide world I stand alone, and think
Till love and fame to nothingness do sink.

—John Keats, *When I have Fears*

On September 30, 2014, Thomas Eric Duncan checked himself into Pres-
byterian Hospital in Dallas, Texas; he was admitted and diagnosed with
Ebola Hemorrhagic Fever. His diagnosis spurred a first world–wide panic.

While a fairly large contingency of Americans, apprised of the surprisingly *un*virulent nature of the pathogen, maintained composure and urged others to do so in the face of a very unlikely pandemic event, many responded rather predictably in the face of threatened plague, demanding closed borders and castigating Duncan for traveling after knowingly coming into contact with actively infected Ebola patients in his hometown in Liberia.

I happened to live less than a mile away from the hospital where Duncan ultimately died, and while I found the level of calm maintained by some Americans laudable, I was ultimately troubled throughout the "Dallas Ebola Outbreak" (which included some three infections) by the purely epidemiological rhetoric mainly used to urge social composure. It is true, of course, that Ebola is neither an airborne nor a fecal-oral disease, but functions rather like a sexually transmitted disease in that it requires contact between the bodily fluids of an infected individual and some orifice or wound of the new host. This certainly does make Ebola of much less concern than any number of droplet-borne infections in circulation at any given time, for we are in less control of the air we breathe than of the foreign blood that enters our bodies.

However, my concern in the face of rampant social media productions explaining these facts in an effort to stem the tide of hysteria was the *lack* of focus on the social factors that had also contributed to Ebola's frightening legacy. Certainly the hemorrhagic nature of the disease is a frightening—if very uncommon—symptom. However, its terrifying and rapid spread in Africa no doubt played a part in the social hysteria in America. The problem I saw with the calming epidemiological explanations put forth in news and social media was the complete absence of discussion of *non*biological factors, such as access to care and postcolonial legacies, that allowed for Ebola's spread in Africa and made it so simple to stymie in America.[1] A simple pair of gloves is often enough to prevent infection with the virus, for instance, yet this "simple" precaution is often an impossibility in Africa, where funds and health resources are famously scarce.

Many humanitarian workers noted African burial practices as responsible for a large portion of the disease transmission, but what about other interpersonal factors? While the government of Liberia publicly announced that it would prosecute Duncan for lying about his exposure to Ebola, and as Americans decried his actions likewise, the fact that his "exposure" involved helping a sick, pregnant neighbor into a taxi to the hospital appeared but as a rather muted murmur in media lines. Newsfeeds also generally underplayed or treated as trivial Duncan's motivations in crossing American borders after this humanitarian effort: he wanted to see his long-term partner and son. The Dallas family lived in a small apartment complex that idled in constant disrepair behind a popular bookstore and across the highway from a shopping mall that caters to some of Dallas's most affluent shoppers. There, Duncan stayed with his family for some time, apparently content with their crowded arrangements when concomitant with the family contact he had so desired.

I have mentioned that seemingly trivial health care equipment such as gloves could mean the difference between sickness and health in regard to Ebola; it will surely be remembered, however, that two of Duncan's nurses contracted the infection in spite of even more advanced contamination protocols. This is partially due to what has now been suspected to be improper training on the part of the hospital, but is also of course due to the fact that the nurses *did* have extended exposure to Duncan's bodily fluids during his active infection. And yet, I would argue that even these seemingly cut-and-dried epidemiological factors have their own social elements. Duncan, Nina Pham, and Amber Vinson all contracted the disease while putting their own fears of contamination aside in order to help a sick member of their community. Some African communities in fact call Ebola "the caretakers' disease," and the idea that this name would be markedly less threatening than its currently very foreign-sounding name has been noted.[2] Even the calmest of legislative reactions to the threat of this supposedly foreign disease involved no less than carting away the entirety of the household belongings of the infected, which were loaded into blue plastic tubs, put onto supposedly sealed containment trucks (which appeared to be normal shipping trucks with "biohazard" labels pasted on the side), and shipped to the Texas coast for incineration (see Figures C.1 and C.2 on page 210).[3] This "decontamination" process was nonnegotiable; patients had no say in the loss of their belongings, for the procedure was mandated by local governments. In the Introduction to this project, I cited David Barnes's inclusion of a late-nineteenth-century Parisian pamphlet describing a similar process for "decontaminating" a home after infectious illness, a process that likewise involved ruining a large portion of the resident's belongings. Figure C.3 on page 211 shows a Victorian decontamination crew such as those mentioned by Barnes, using nineteenth-century travel and containment mechanisms, which nevertheless look strikingly similar to the equipment used in 2014.[4] My analysis of this process questioned the notion that disease could ever be fully contained or purified. On a more practical level, I expressed doubt in my introduction that the necessary hermetically sealed containers and such existed in the nineteenth century. However, the notion

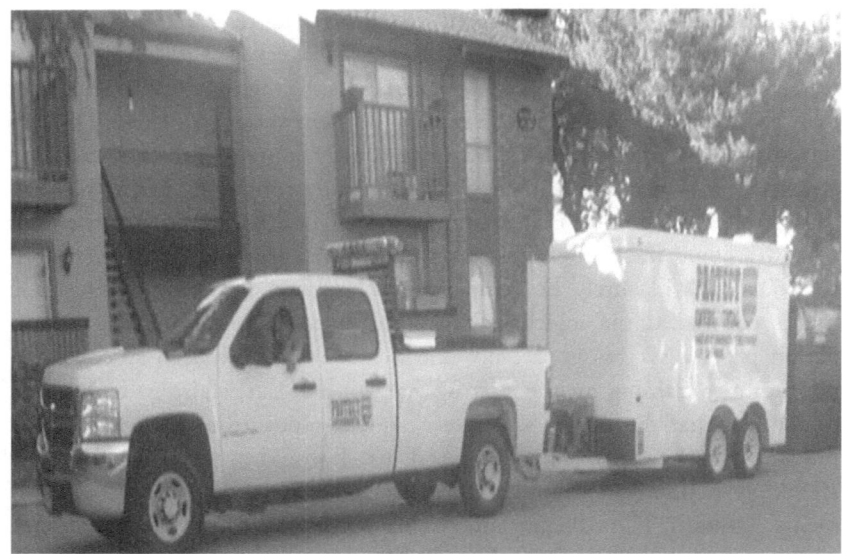

Figure C.1. Decontamination Crew in Dallas, TX, 2014.

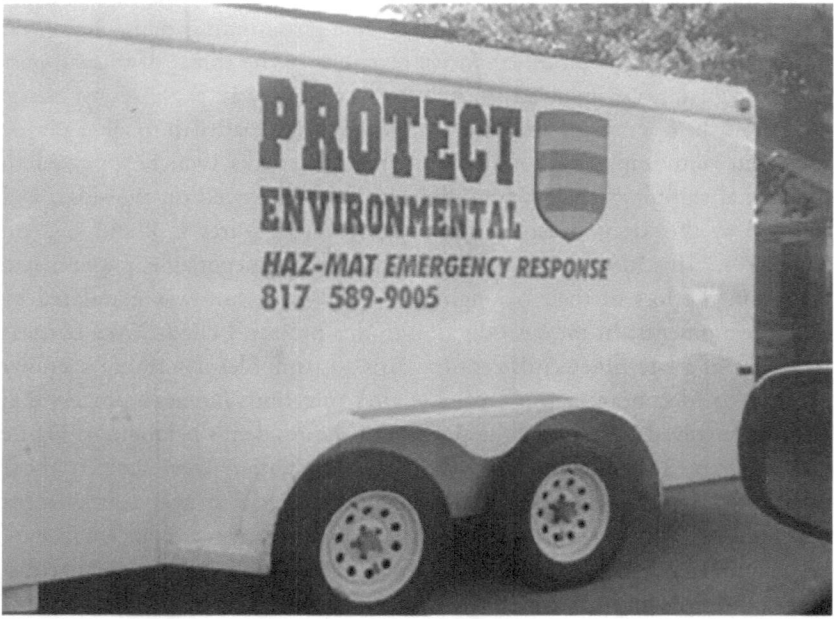

Figure C.2. Decontamination Crew in Dallas, TX, 2014.

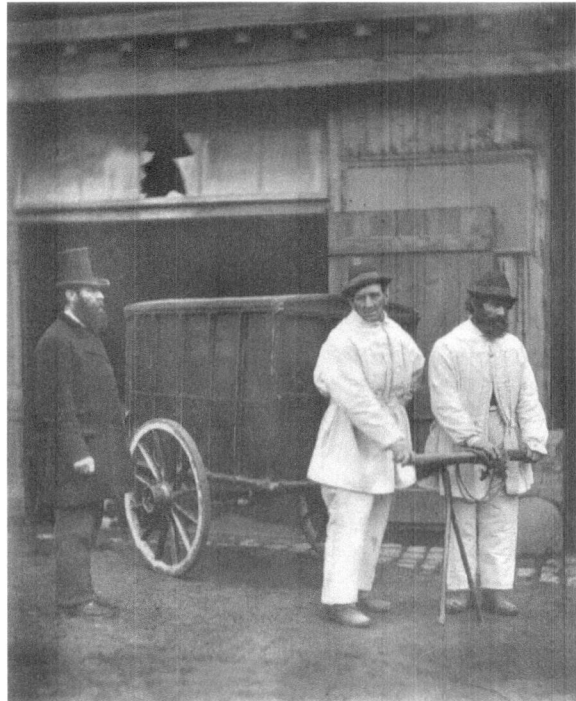

Figure C.3. Decontamination Crew in London, 1877.

of perfectly attainable purity clearly remains with us, for our processes for fully purifying the homes of contagious individuals differ quite little today from those employed in the late nineteenth century, and today's plastic bins and standard moving trucks used to collect the infected belongings hardly seem more capable of containing microscopic contaminants. Obviously, it is the imagined *sense* of purity at issue here, and one might almost assume these efforts were made to calm public fervor rather than for their potential to effect any real change in the microbial particles still present in the carpets and walls of the patients' homes, along with the trucks themselves. Even today, then, the dilemma of human contact in the face of disease is quite palpable. Duncan died because of his commitment to helping a neighbor in need, and he infected two others because of his desire to be near those he loved most. Are there morally clear decisions in this Petri dish of human experience, emotion, and infectious particles? Possibly not.

But this sociophysical cocktail, complete with all its moral ambiguity, is a fundamentally intrinsic part of disease—of the human experience—as I see it, even today. Western society has not, I think, moved much past the questions tentatively raised by the Victorians in their first encounters with the new worldviews provided by germ theory. If anything, I would suggest that the recent past has seen a backpedaling from their thoughtful ethical considerations because, much as many late-nineteenth-century authors seemed to fear, scientific "fact" has become a new sort of Godhead, and thus modern motivation to resist neoliberal biopolitics is therefore next to none. "Scientific fact" is now so little questioned in the public realm that its findings tend to take precedence over the humanitarian and deep, raw, interpersonal concerns we might be left with if divested of these ostensibly infallible truth claims. Even when these facts appear incontrovertible, I argue that the Victorians were astutely "onto something" in their sense that inarguable facts do not necessarily reveal the path to human (and by that I mean human*itarian*) progress.

Grant Allen's social imperative, mentioned in chapter 5, that "no unit can wholly sever itself from the social organism of which it is a corpuscle" begs readers quite passionately, I think, to be open to risk encounters that could, in fact, be vivifying for us.[5] Because of the rather indirect role infectious disease plays in that novel on a literal level, I have chosen not to devote an entire body chapter to the text. However, its metaphoric reliance on notions of contamination and contagion provides an apt point of reflection for these closing pages. Grant's admonition, I believe, is on one level a statement of fact in the modern, globalized world with which the Victorians were already faced. Further, it is a veritable jeremiad, warning of the consequences of attempts to believe and act as if the opposite were true, a point to which I will return directly. Part of the hysterical reaction to Duncan's mere presence in America, I would like to suggest, has to do with the breaking down of our illusory sense that anyone *can* live separately from our fellow man in a world where jet travel (or, just as effective for disease transmission in the Victorian era, boat travel) paired with disease renders the permeability of our cutaneous membranes all too obvious. As Kristeva so poetically puts it:

> How can I be without border? That elsewhere that I imagine beyond the present, or that I hallucinate so that I might, in a present time, speak to you, conceive of you—it is now here,

jetted, abjected, into "my" world. . . . I behold the breaking down of a world that has erased its borders.[6]

As seen in the introduction, all of us rely on a belief in our ability to exist independently of others and on our capability to define ourselves against others for our maintenance of a sense of selfhood—an ability to exist without risk encounters, that is. Disease destabilizes all of this hard-won existential stability, however. When entire communities and not simply individuals are involved, such as in the feared spread of Ebola, the stakes are necessarily much higher, involving questions of identity, both national and individual, a dynamic that was similarly explored in the introduction. But these connections, as Grant insists, exist, for better or worse. Africa's outbreak is everyone's outbreak—or threatens to be, however convenient it might be to look the other way and pretend otherwise. This, I believe, is the source of the 2014 Ebola Hysteria, the labeling as an American epidemic what was in fact only a triparty infection. The disease had dared to cross a borders where citizens believed themselves to be beyond the pale of such infections, and the startling revelation that our repressed fears, so neatly (and imaginarily) ensconced in another continent, could return to haunt us, was overpowering. Kristeva again puts the matter poignantly:

> The abject has only one quality of the object—that of being opposed to *I* . . . the object, however, through its opposition, settles me within the fragile texture of a desire for meaning, which, as a matter of fact, makes me ceaselessly and infinitely homologous to it. . . . It lies outside, beyond the set, and does not seem to agree to the latter's rules of the game. And yet, from its place of banishment, the abject does not cease challenging its master.[7]

The 2012 West Nile "outbreak" in North Dallas revealed similar fears and perhaps even more frenzied attempts to eject awareness of them.[8] Although the so-called outbreak resulted in fewer deaths than the seasonal flu, aerial pesticide sprayings continue to this day, physically marking the attempts to deny that diseases of the "other" were now part of this community, as well. The virus's omnipresence was palpable as the rising (but fairly few) death tolls were ticked off daily, summarily, and perfunctorily on the local news. The thrum of low-flying planes spraying pesticides below the tree line punctuated the summer nights. Automated text messages sent from local news stations illuminated cell phone screens across the city, warning citizens to remain indoors while the poisonous fumes were dispersed just above their rooftops. The widespread sense of contamination remained palpable even after the sprayings, as the ground became littered with the bodies of dazed and dying insects (mostly not mosquitoes) that had succumbed to the poison—casualties, one might say, of this war on West Nile Terror. In the days after and even in between the weeks of nightly sprayings, however, the resilient mosquitoes continued to hover about. The feeble crescendoing twang of their thirsty song wafted in the air, a remnant of man's most recent attempt to elude the death and disease deemed so out of place in affluent, white America. The city seemed united amid the backdrop of mosquitos' hums. Everyone, in a body, seemed to imagine the virus in the mosquitos' bellies—the penetration of their proboscises—and shudder. The convulsing bodies of bees and the crackling crunch of cicadas dying underfoot filled the campus of Southern Methodist University where I was writing this study, and I was reminded of the subtle note of warning in Allen's words: we can*not* separate ourselves from the interstitial tissue of the world around us. And what if we try? I stared at a wasp crawling in palsied lurches on the sidewalk before me as I contemplated the answer to this question.

Of course, as is clear in light of the previous chapters, I intend these examples not simply to illustrate the ways that disease frightens us and catalyzes our retreat into an imagined membranous bubble of safety, but also the endlessly multifaceted ways in which disease shapes our world and forces us to consider our connection to the organisms around us. Priscilla Wald has claimed that disease can define communities by uniting groups of peoples in a shared, pressure-cooker sense of threat during a contagious outbreak. But disease itself is often identified at the borders of what is already recognized as a community—after all, it is interesting that the disease involved in the 2012 Texas outbreak will probably never be called North Dallas Virus. No, white, Western privilege cannot seem to phenomenologically sustain the notion that this disease could define its community. Likewise, Ebola will certainly never be renamed Caretakers' Disease, for this implicit identification of *unwilling* caretakers would threaten perhaps more than the disease itself.

Indeed, as Anne Finger would have it, the very notion of an "epidemic" is based on varying groups' relationships to disease. She has pointed out, for example, that polio was not considered an epidemic illness—in spite of being in fact endemic to most nations and peoples throughout history—until it affected a middle-class white America that had considered itself beyond the pale of infectious diseases.[9] I would argue that Ebola and West Nile were, similarly, not considered meaningful outbreaks until they dared to confront Americans with not only their undeniable interconnection to the rest of the environmental and social world, but also with the consequences of having so long attempted to deny such connections. Perhaps "Africa's outbreak" would not have come to the United States if better attempts had been made to aid Africa in its fight against the epidemic. Instead, before Duncan's arrival, and arguably after it, the United States indulged in the first-world delusion that it could stay safely ensconced, and that disease would not penetrate its borders. Our attempts to exterminate absolutely all the vectors of West Nile with poison illustrated rather vividly, to my mind, the consequences of our determined efforts to maintain a sense of these illusory borders. It does not take an entomologist, after all, to know that the ecosystem—insects included—hangs in delicate balance, and that vast extermination of local insects bodes ill for the future of our biome. No, we cannot separate ourselves from the vast world of which we are a part, and our attempts to do so seem to wreak more havoc than they prevent.

The trajectory of Allen's novel illustrates his likely answer to the question raised earlier: "What if we try anyway"? Herminia Barton, the novel's protagonist, is determined to live with the man she loves openly and outside of marriage, in a very purposeful attempt to flout social convention and begin a revolution to change the moral status quo of the day. I have explored similar dynamics in chapter 2 as evidence of authorial approval of existing outside of a tainted moral system. However, Allen's novel suggests that Herminia's sense that she can live in complete isolation from what she views as a morally tainted society is misguided. After her partner dies of typhoid fever—a disease the Victorians considered to be one of filth and contamination itself—she is left destitute with her young daughter Dolores, whom she raises in isolation with plans to educate the child to be exactly like herself. Much to Herminia's dismay, Dolores in fact *wants* to be a part of the social amalgam, and in this manner rebels against her mother's sense of morally righteous nonconformity. Alone and faced with her failed attempts to control and isolate her daughter, albeit for an ostensibly good cause, Herminia commits suicide at the novel's conclusion.

While the attempt to live outside stifling moral norms is presented quite positively in Hardy's *The Woodlanders* (as seen in chapter 2), the characters in this novel nevertheless reunite with one another on their new moral path and return to join the community, renewed in their ethical and marital drives *within* it. Conversely, the Alving family in *Ghosts* virtually withers away by the play's conclusion because of Mrs. Alving's continued determination to live in moral superiority to those around her. Allen's novel indicates that whatever the aim, attempted moral isolation is not only contradictory (for what are morals if not defined in part based on community interactions?), but damning. Allen incorporates typhoid fever into his novel, a disease seldom seen in Victorian novels because of its direct association with fecal matter and bodily bile. I argue that this constitutes a direct and almost crass statement on Allen's part illustrating that Herminia's ostensibly morally pure family is tainted from within by her persistent belief that isolated existence is both possible and preferable to a life of interaction with her fellow man. Moreover, even after her partner's death, the words *contagion, contamination,* and *taint* appear more in *The Woman Who Did* than perhaps any other novel of the century. For instance, the narrator, describes Herminia's isolated employment as a freelance author and claims that that field had been freed from "the leprous taint of that national moral blight that calls itself 'respectability.' "[10] Later, when Dolores's grandfather meets her in the street and gives her a coin, Herminia "caught her child up with a cry of terror; and that very same evening, she changed the tainted sovereign with Dolly for another one."[11] She then pens a warning note to her would-be father-in-law, instructing him that her daughter is to be "kept from all contagions" of this kind.[12] In spite of the seemingly small role that disease plays in this novel, then, I argue that Allen's claims clearly—in light of my arguments in this project thus far—associate social isolation with imperatives surrounding microbial purity which were so common at this time. One 1899 article describes the attitudes surrounding disease thus:

> All germs were at once denounced as harmful, and sterilization of everything, even to coins and clothing, became the order of the day. But [then] it was found, to our dismay, that not merely our food, the air we breathe, the soil we live on, but even the surface and cavities of our own bodies, skin, hair, mouth, and stomach swarmed with bacteria.[13]

Moreover, I argue that Allen's warning, along with those of his contemporaries, are voices necessary to attend to even today, for disease remains a given even in our antibiotic, antiviral age. The more we would like to insist that cancers and hypertensive conditions are of greater seriousness or prevalence than these supposedly vitiated infective illnesses, the more, I maintain, we demonstrate our *disconnection* from the world around us, where infection is relegated to less prosperous countries—imaginatively, at least. This logic conveniently sidesteps recognition of the rampant staphylococcus and streptococcus infections that are rather endemic to hospital environments, which necessitates a further sidestepping awareness of the immunosuppressed individuals—cancer patients, diabetic patients, and the like—who are most prone to these infections. The sense that infectious disease is no longer threatening, then, reveals no less than the sense that some people can live safely in the epicenter of a somehow privileged, purified world, while sickened individuals are shuffled to its margins.

In a perverse twist of this dynamic, the antivaccine movement demonstrates just this flippant attitude in the face of diseases that once decimated populations. There is something rather antisocial in the sense that one can live within a population and not be affected by its endemic pathogens. It would, of course, be possible to read this dynamic in just the opposite way: as embodying the willingness to embrace the "messy" side of human experience that I have mentioned in my introduction. However, and this is perhaps the point I want to drive home the most in these final pages, this "messy" engagement with the biosocial amalgam of humanity is *not* about a *desire* for *disease,* but about a desire to engage with the human community that takes precedence over other, baser fears. Thus, I interpret the antivaccine movement as yet another example of a contemporary sense that anyone can somehow live in isolation from the broad, organic world—human and viral—around us, and that humans can somehow ignore their responsibility to and necessary, unavoidable interconnection with the vast wealth of life in which we all live in wondrous symbiosis. Recently, autistic authors have spoken out against the antivaccine movement, citing its underlying stigma against cognitive alterities. This stigma, they argue, is so great that physical death seems preferable to a nonnormative mental state.[16] Here again, I note a decided tone of isolationist superiority in the antivaccine movement, which physically imagines itself apart from the biological community it exists within and simultaneously so far beyond the reach of infectious disease (a problematic viewpoint, which I have covered already) that it has moved beyond Victorian-style fears of infection to fears of mental disease. Like *fin-de-siècle* insistence on physical purity, the antivaccine movement as I see it recoils so viscerally from mental "impurity," that it opts to take on the risk of physical contamination. As I have suggested earlier, the willingness to take this risk implies nothing short of a complete sense that this contamination will never occur via herd immunity—that is, protection from the very social group they envision themselves as physically and spiritually set apart from.

Disease is a part of life. I would venture to assert, as I have attempted to do through the previous pages, that it is a vital part of the human experience. And while no one ever desires to contract a disease, I nevertheless find, as I believe a handful of late Victorian authors found before me, that the presence of a disease can nevertheless tell us a lot about the vitalizing effects of engaged existence in the human and animal community of which we are a part. Their works demonstrate this to readers, inviting them to cautiously reapproach the risky engagement with this potentially contaminated community. Their novels urge readers to dip their toes into the humanitarian realm of deep human connection in a world too much ruled by scientific mandates. Certainly, contact with a virally infected pregnant woman, a bite from an infected mosquito, or surface contact with the salmonella germs that cause typhoid may result in disease. These are factual possibilities. But the value of connecting with a dying woman in her last moments or of accepting the risks inherent in our natural environment cannot be quantitatively calculated. As the Victorians discovered, disease is all around us, potentially lurking in every moment of mindful contact with our social and vegetable world; and the insistent subtextual admonition of the authors I have highlighted here is: "This vitalizing contact is worth the risk." As Thomas Duncan has shown, as diseased mosquitos have made clear, and as Allen demonstrated 120 years ago, we can never be, never are—are spiritually *de*vitalized when attempting to be—"kept from all contagion."

Notes

Introduction

1. "The Germ Theory Again," *Chambers's Journal of Popular Literature, Science, and Art*, November 1897; titular emphasis mine.

2. "Vegetable Villains," *Good Words*, December 1883, 730–31.

3. Ibid., 730.

4. Ibid.

5. Ibid., 731.

6. Ibid.

7. Julia Kristeva, *Powers of Horror* (New York: Columbia University Press, 1982), 3.

8. Ibid.

9. Benedict Anderson, *Imagined Communities* (London: Verso, 1983), 4.

10. Giorgio Agamben, *Homo Sacer: Sovereign Power and Bare Life* (Stanford: Stanford University Press, 1995), 6.

11. See, for instance, the special issue *Rethinking the Reception of the Germ Theory of Disease* in *The Journal of the History of Medicine* 52 (1997).

12. Miriam Bailin has addressed the potential of the Victorian sickroom for evoking this sense of wholeness through the vessel of disease. Miriam Bailin, *The Sickroom in Victorian Fiction: The Art of Being Ill* (Cambridge: Cambridge University Press, 1994).

13. Thomas Postlewait, *Prophet of the New Drama: William Archer and the Ibsen Campaign* (Westport: Greenwood, 1985), 3.

14. For the purposes of this project, I use the term *Victorian* to apply to Norwegian and British cultures during the late nineteenth century, so similar are the cultural zeitgeists that Ibsen and Hardy, among others, claimed to be writing against.

15. J. V. Chapple, *Science and Literature in the Nineteenth Century* (Hampshire: Macmillan, 1986), 1.

16. John H. Cartwright, "Those Dreadful Hammers: Geology and Evolution in Nineteenth-Century Literature," in *Literature and Science: Social Impact and Interaction*, ed. John H. Cartwright and Brian Baker (Santa Barbara: ABC-CLIO, 2005), 175.

17. Richard D. Altick, *Victorian People and Ideas: A Companion for the Modern Reader of Victorian Literature* (New York: Norton, 1974), 99.

18. Ibid.

19. Qtd. in Zimmerman and taken from the *Quarterly Review*, 1827. Virginia Zimmerman, *Excavating Victorians* (Albany: State University of New York Press, 2008), 1.

20. Thomas Hardy, *A Pair of Blue Eyes* (Hertfordshire: Wordsworth Classics, 1995), 172.

21. Altick, *Victorian People and Ideas*, 99; Cartwright, "Those Dreadful Hammers," 175; Pamela Gossin, *Thomas Hardy's Novel Universe: Astronomy, Cosmology, and Gender in the Post-Darwinian World* (Aldershot: Ashgate, 2007), 80.

22. Cartwright, "Those Dreadful Hammers," 175.

23. Altick, *Victorian People and Ideas*, 111; Brian Baker, "From Entropy to Chaos," in *Literature and Science: Social Impact and Interaction*, ed. John H. Cartwright and Brian Baker (Santa Barbara: ABC-CLIO, 2005), 245; Chapple, *Science and Literature*, 46.

24. Ibid., 82; Aiyleen Fyfe and Bernard Lightman, eds., *Science in the Marketplace: Nineteenth-Century Sites and Experiences* (Chicago: University of Chicago Press, 2007), 3.

25. Gossin, *Hardy's Novel Universe*, 82.

26. Ibid., 83.

27. Anne DeWitt, " 'The Actual Sky Is a Horror': Thomas Hardy and the Arnoldian Conception of Science," *Nineteenth-Century Literature* 61, no. 4 (2007): 480–81.

28. Thomas Hardy, *Two on a Tower* (New York: Penguin, 1999), 57–58.

29. J. Hillis Miller, *The Disappearance of God: Five Nineteenth-Century Writers* (Cambridge: Harvard University Press, 1963).

30. Ibid., 2.

31. Matthew Arnold, "Stanzas from the Grand Chartreuse," 85–86.

32. George Levine, *Realism, Ethics, and Secularism: Essays on Victorian Literature and Science* (Cambridge: Cambridge University Press, 2008), 3.

33. Ibid., 110.

34. Ignaz Semmelweis, *The Etiology, Concept, and Prophylaxis of Childbed Fever*, ed. Sherwin B. Nuland and Ferenc A. Gyorgyey (Birmingham: The Classics of Medicine Library, 1981).

35. Oliver Wendell Holmes, "The Contagiousness of Pueperal Fever," in *The Writings of Oliver Wendell Holmes In Thirteen Volumes*. Volume IX (Cambridge: Riverside Press, 1892).

36. For more on Lister, see Terrie M. Romano, "The Cattle Plague of 1865 and the Reception of 'The Germ Theory' in Mid-Victorian Britain," *Journal of the History of Medicine* 52 (1997).

37. W. F. Bynum, *Science and the Practice of Medicine in the Nineteenth Century* (Cambridge: Cambridge University Press, 1994), 127–29; Otis, *Membranes*, 25–31.

38. Paul De Kruif, qtd. in Otis, *Membranes*, 5.

39. "The Battle of the Bacilli," *The Outlook*, December 30, 1899, 713.

40. W. B. Carpenter, "The Germ-Theory of Zymotic Diseases: Considered from the Natural History Point of View," in *The Nineteenth-Century: A Monthly Review* (February 1884): 318.

41. J. Anderson Smith, "Immunity from Disease," *The Wesleyan-Methodist Magazine*, June 1893, 454.

42. "Another Book on Bacteriology," *The Saturday Review*, August 1, 1891, 144.

43. Otis, *Membranes*, 4.

44. Ibid., 5.

45. Ibid., 31–35.

46. Ibid., 21.

47. Qtd. in Anne McWhir, "Mary Shelley's Anti-Contagionism: *The Last Man* as 'Fatal Narrative," *Mosaic: An Interdisciplinary Critical Journal* 35, no. 2 (2002).

48. Otis, *Membranes*, 5.

49. David Barnes, *Great Stink of Paris* (Baltimore: Johns Hopkins University Press, 2006), 2. Bruno Latour has also discussed germ theory as a non-innovation in *The Pasteurization of France*.

50. Ibid., 3.

51. Levine, *Realism, Ethics, and Secularism*, vi.

52. Barnes, *Great Stink of Paris*, 147; emphasis mine.

53. Ibid.

54. Ibid., 148.

55. Ibid., 144.

56. Ibid., 147.

57. Ibid., 150.

58. Ibid.

59. "Successful Disinfectant," in *Medical and Other Uses of Carbolic Acid* (Manchester: F. C. Calvert).

60. W. C., "The Germ Theory," *Chambers's Journal of Popular Literature, Science, and Art*, March 4, 1876, 147.

61. Helen W. Bissell, "Health, Beauty, and the Toilet," *Bow Bells*, August 19, 1892, 178.

62. Ibid.

63. Izal Powder Advertisement, *Strand Magazine*, January 1893, xvi.

64. Ibid.

65. Advertisement for Eno's Fruit Salt, *Longman's Magazine*, November 1897, 674.

66. Ibid.

67. Advertisement for Clarke's Blood Mixture, *The Gentleman's Magazine*, December 1896, 4.

68. Advertisement for the Carbolic Smoke Ball, *Tinsleys' Magazine*, July 1889, 137, and Wellcome images, "Carbolic Smoke Ball," 1890.

69. Advertisement for Eno's Fruit Salt, *Strand Magazine*, January 1892, 19.

70. Vapo-Cresolene Vaporizer, product box.

71. Barnes, *Great Stink of Paris*, 2.

72. Ibid., 146.

Chapter 1. Keep Bleeding

1. W. B. Carpenter, "The Germ-Theory of Zymotic Diseases: Considered from the Natural History Point of View," *The Nineteenth-Century: A Monthly Review* (Feb. 1884): 317.

2. Rajani Sudan has detailed productively the modes via which this in fact ancient techne was transported from Eastern cultures to Western ones, and then labeled as Western via nominal changes (such as "inoculation" being changed to "vaccination"). For more information, see her book *Alchemy and Empire*.

3. For further reading on this topic, see Sudan, who speaks a great deal to this complex interplay of xenophobia, a sense of otherness versus selfhood, and borders. Rajani Sudan, *Fair Exotics: Xenophobic Subjects in English Literature, 1720–1850* (Philadelphia: University of Pennsylvania Press, 2002).

4. Daniel Defoe, *Journal of the Plague Year* (Oxford: Oxford University Press, 1998), 56.

5. Ibid.

6. Priscilla Wald, *Contagious: Cultures, Carriers, and the Outbreak Narrative* (Durham: Duke University Press, 2008), 2.

7. Jennifer Cooke, "Writing Plague: Transforming Narrative, Witnessing, and History," in *The Tapestry of Health, Illness, and Disease*, ed. Peter L Twohig and Vera Kalitzkus (Amsterdam: Rodopi, 2008), 22.

8. Julia Kristeva, *Powers of Horror: An Essay on Abjection* (New York: Columbia University Press, 1982), 3.

9. Ibid., 3. William Ian Miller notes, "What disgusts is the capacity for life, and *not* just because life implies its correlative death and decay . . . [but because] images of decay imperceptibly slide into images of fertility and out again." William Ian Miller, *The Anatomy of Disgust* (Cambridge: Harvard University Press, 1997), 40; emphasis mine.

10. J. F. D. Shrewsbury, *A History of the Bubonic Plague in the British Isles* (Cambridge: Harvard University Press, 1970), 5. Although the plague is largely transmitted through flea bites, fear of the leaking, pus-filled sores associated with

the plague can hardly be overstated, particularly in the context of a pre-germ-theory society. See Shrewsbury, *History of the Bubonic Plague*, 5.

11. I have derived this term from a concept Wald calls "communicability configuring community." Wald, *Contagious*, 12.

12. Daniel Defoe, *Due Preparations for the Plague, as for Soul as Body* (London: J. M. Dent, 1895), 81.

13. Defoe, *Journal*, 76.

14. Ibid., 81–82.

15. Ibid., 172.

16. Ibid., 81. It must be noted here that contemporary medical practice *did* hold that suppurated sores implied a greater chance of survival, a fact it would be remiss to ignore in analyzing the portrayal of doctors' attempts at their perforation. Defoe himself notes this in *A Journal*, writing that "if these Swellings could be brought to a Head, and to break and run . . . the Patient generally recover'd; whereas those, who . . . were struck with Death at the Beginning, and had the Tokens come out upon them, often went about indifferent easy, till a little before they died." Ibid., 82. This is, in fact, a contemporary misunderstanding of the fact that if the patient's buboes suppurate, they have simply made it past the usual course of infection during which death is *most likely*. That is, death often occurs before suppuration can take place; see Shrewsbury, *Bubonic Plague*, 5. Defoe's own words interestingly and unconsciously belie this reality. In spite of the contemporary medical reasoning behind these attempts at suppuration, the fact remains that Defoe repeatedly depicts such acts and treats them with a high degree of angst and determination.

17. George Childs Kohn, ed., *Encyclopedia of Plague and Pestilence: From Ancient Times to the Present*, 3rd ed. (New York: Facts on File, 2008), 234.

18. Ibid.

19. Katherine E. Ellison, *Fatal News: Reading and Information Overload in Early Eighteenth-Century Literature* (New York: Routledge, 2006), 91.

20. Wald, *Contagious*, 53–54.

21. Nadja Durbach has helpfully elucidated the sociopolitical factors underlying the vaccination debates in England beginning in this period. For more information, see Nadja Durbach, *Bodily Matters* (Durham: Duke University Press, 2006).

25. William Douglass, *A Dissertation Concerning Inoculation of the Small-Pox* (Boston: Henchman, 1730).

23. Ibid.

24. Legard Sparham, *Reasons Against the Practice of Inoculating the Small-Pox* (London: Peele, 1722), 10–11.

25. Ibid., 23.

26. W. Wagstaffe, *A Letter To Dr. Friend Shewing the Danger and Uncertainity of Inoculating the Small-Pox* (London: Butler, 1722), 10–11.

27. Ibid., 11.

28. Shrewsbury, *Bubonic Plague,* 6.

29. Wald points out that "the use of disease to imagine as well as regulate communities powerfully enacts the most anxious dimensions of national relatedness." Wald, *Contagious,* 67.

30. Defoe, *Journal,* 94.

31. Ibid., 94–95.

32. Defoe's merchant-class roots are well known. See Ian A. Bell, *Defoe's Fiction* (London: Croom Helm, 1985), 15; John J. Richetti, *Daniel Defoe* (Boston: Twayne, 1987), 1.

33. Bram Dijkstra, *Defoe and Economics: The Fortunes of Roxana in the History of Interpretation* (New York: St. Martin's, 1987), 11.

34. Ibid., 6.

35. Wald, *Contagious,* 2.

36. Brodsley argues that Defoe situates "each public health action . . . within a complex web of factors" to illustrate the array of interactions that affect public policy. Laurel Brodsley, "Defoe's *Journal of the Plague Year:* A Model for Stories of Plagues," in *AIDS: The Literary Response,* ed. Emmanual S. Nelson (New York: Twayne, 1992), 13.

37. Critics have made different uses of these data, and discussion of the connection between bubonic "tokens" and currency appears in a number of articles, including Armstrong and Tennenhouse, among others. Nancy Armstrong and Leonard Tennenhouse, "Sovereignty and the Form of Formlessness," *Differences: A Journal of Feminist Cultural Studies* 20, no. 2–3 (2009): 148–78.

38. Daniel Defoe, *Compleat English Tradesman* (London, 1726), II.9; emphasis added. Thomas Keith Meier also notes this passage for its discussion of Defoe's emphasis on trade. Thomas Keith Meier, *Defoe and the Defense of Commerce* (Victoria: University of Victoria Press, 1987), 42.

39. Ibid., 42.

40. Ibid.

41. William James Roosen, *Daniel Defoe and Diplomacy* (Selinsgrove: Susquehanna University Press, 1986), 77.

42. Ibid., 76.

43. Dijkstra, *Defoe and Economics,* 42–43.

44. See Armstrong and Tennenhouse for their commentary on Defoe's use of the body politic.

45. Defoe, *Compleat English Tradesman,* qtd. in Dijkstra, *Defoe and Economics,* 8.

46. Ibid., 9.

47. Dijkstra, *Defoe and Economics,* 33.

48. See David Trotter, *Circulation: Defoe, Dickens, and the Economies of the Novel* (New York: St. Martins, 1988), 61–63.

49. Qtd. in Trotter, *Circulation*, 62.

50. Ibid.

51. Trotter, *Circulation*, 56. In *Defoe and Economics*, Dijkstra details in great length the contemporary metaphors of the pond versus the spring (the former stagnates and fails to reproduce, and the latter proliferates and feeds many other bodies) to similar ends.

52. Defoe, *Compleat English Tradesman*, II.10.

53. Ibid.

54. Harris has made similar claims about the characterization of the body politic in the early modern period. Asserting that the metaphor of the body politic was so powerful that other concerns about the state were also figured in corporeal terms, he argues, for instance, that many authors suggested that "every component or function of the body—even its most noxious or toxic elements, even pathogenic foreign bodies that have infiltrated it—contributes to its health." Jonathan Gil Harris, *Foreign Bodies and the Body Politic: Discourses of Social Pathology in Early Modern England* (Cambridge, Cambridge University Press, 1998), 49.

55. Defoe, *Due Preparations*, 10.

56. Ibid., 10–11.

57. Critics are generally aware of the fact that Defoe's authorship was largely for hire, as any perusal of his biography evinces. Brodsley notes that his specific work on *A Journal*, and certainly, it must be granted, *Due Preparations* as well, was "part of a larger public education program developed . . . to prepare the British for the bubonic plague" (12), a point that Margaret Healy has also noted. Brodsley, "Defoe's *Journal*," 12; Margaret Healy, "Defoe's *Journal* and the English Plague Writing Tradition," *Literature and Medicine* 22, no. 1 (2003). More specifically, Ellison notes that these two texts were likely written in specific support of Walpole's Quarantine Act; Ellison, *Fatal News*, 91.

58. Defoe, *Due Preparations*, 10.

59. Defoe, *Journal*, 215.

60. Defoe, *Due Preparations*, 15.

61. Brodsley, "Defoe's *Journal*," 16.

62. Defoe, *Journal*, 70.

63. Defoe, *Due Preparations*, 15–16.

64. Ibid., 50.

65. Ibid., 56.

66. Ibid., 48–49.

67. Ibid., 56.

68. In fact, while the man and his family never contract the plague, they do suffer from a disease of a "scorbutic" nature, which Defoe ascribes to their "want of air for breath" (Defoe, *Due Preparations*, 67), which is, of course, a result of their confinement. Interestingly, while Defoe sets the patriarch of this family up as an exemplar of successfully regulated flow of goods and contact with the outer world,

he falters only in his overly meticulous mediation of this interaction. Though the family survives the plague, they develop a festering disease of the individual body that eats away at corporeal membranes from the inside out. Defoe seems to suggest here that one could err on the side of *too much* access, which, while dangerous, allows for life-giving circulation.

69. Alan Bewell, *Romanticism and Colonial Disease* (Baltimore: Johns Hopkins University Press, 1999), 296.

70. Ibid.

71. Ibid.

72. Mary Shelley, *The Last Man* (Hertfordshire: Wordsworth Classics, 2004), 175; 340.

73. Ibid., 206.

74. Ibid., 184.

75. Ibid.

76. Ibid., 186.

77. Ibid.

78. Bewell, 303.

79. Shelley, *Last Man*, 199.

80. Ibid., 208.

81. Ibid., 179.

82. Ibid., 174.

83. George Childs Kohn, ed., *Encyclopedia of Plague and Pestilence,* 3rd ed. (New York: Facts on File), 51.

84. William Woodville, *Reports of a Series of Inoculations for the Variolæ Vaccine or Cow-pox* (London: James Phillips and Son, 1799).

85. Shelley, *Last Man*, 241.

86. Ibid.

87. Ibid.

88. Ibid., 204.

89. Ibid., 203–204.

90. Ibid., 216.

91. Alan Bewell, while focusing primarily on the colonial aspects of this encounter, also terms this as "inoculation." Bewell, *Romanticism*, 313.

92. Shelley, *Last Man*, 268.

93. Ibid., 269.

94. Ibid., 204; emphasis mine.

95. Ibid., 229.

96. Ibid.

97. Ibid.

98. Ibid.

99. Ibid.

100. Ibid., 230.

101. Melissa Bailes, "The Psychologization of Geological Catastrophe in Mary Shelley's *The Last Man*," *ELH* 82 (2015): 672.

102. Shelley, *Last Man*, 235.

103. Ibid.

104. Bewell, *Romanticism*, 311.

105. Shelley, *Last Man*, 196.

106. Ibid.

107. Ibid., 196; 206; 340.

108. For debates about the nature of the contagion, see, for example, Anne McWhir, "Mary Shelley's Anti-Contagionism: *The Last Man* as 'Fatal Narrative,'" *Mosaic* 35, no. 2 (2002), and Peter Melville, "The Problem of Immunity in *The Last Man*," *SEL* 47, no. 4 (2007).

109. For Shelley's understanding of contagion, see again McWhir and Mellville.

110. Shelley, *Last Man*, 328.

111. Allan Conrad Christensen, *Nineteenth-Century Narratives of Contagion: "Our Feverish Contact"* (New York: Routledge, 2005), 291.

112. Shelley, *Last Man*, 352.

113. Ibid., 213.

114. Ibid., 368.

115. Ibid.

116. Ibid., 369.

117. Ibid., 368.

118. The retrospective revelation of the death of H. F. is discussed by Armstrong and Tennenhouse, DeGabriele, Ellison, and Seager, among others. Armstrong and Tennenhouse, "Sovreignty"; Peter DeGabriele, "Intimacy, Survival, and Resistance: Daniel Defoe's *A Journal of the Plague Year*," *ELH* 77, no. 1 (2010); Nicholas Seager, "Lies, Damned Lies, and Statistics: Epistemology and Fiction in Defoe's *A Journal of the Plague Year*," *Modern Language Review* 103, no. 3 (2008).

119. Shelley, *Last Man*, 371.

120. Giorgio Agamben, *Homo Sacer: Sovereign Power and Bare Life* (Stanford: Stanford University Press, 1995), 6.

121. Jennifer A. Wagner-Lawlor, "Performing History, Performing Humanity in Mary Shelley's *The Last Man*," *Studies in English Literature* (Autumn 2002): 769.

122. Armstrong and Tennenhouse, "Sovreignty," 170.

123. Ibid.

124. Cynthia Wall, "Novel Streets: The Rebuilding of London and Defoe's *A Journal of the Plague Year*," *Studies in the Novel* 30, no. 2 (1998): 170.

125. Wagner-Lawlor, "Performing History," 772.

126. Shelley, *Last Man*, 174.

Chapter 2. "A Speculative Idea"

1. Numerous scholars of nineteenth-century medicine (including Leavitt, Rooks, and Wertz and Wertz) have noted the importance of this statement as representative of the development of the obstetrical practice in America. Judith Walzer Leavitt, *Brought to Bed: Childbearing in America 1750–1950* (New York: Oxford University Press, 1986); Judith Pence Rooks, *Midwifery and Childbirth in America* (Philadelphia: Temple University Press, 1997); Richard W. Wertz and Dorothy C. Wertz, *Lying-In: A History of Childbirth in America* (New Haven: Yale University Press, 1989).

2. Henry James, *Washington Square* (New York: The Modern Library, 2002), 3.

3. Although Andrew Scheiber has written on *Washington Square* and Darwinian evolution, the novel has yet to be connected to broader scientific discourse of the time. Andrew Scheiber, "The Doctor's Order: Eugenic Anxiety in Henry James's *Washington Square*," *Literature and Medicine* 15, no. 2 (1996).

4. Since bacteriology as a specific field didn't develop until the 1880s and was an integral part of the ultimate solidification of the previously extant germ theory, James sets up *Washington Square* as a retrospective through which he can explore early germ theory culture in America in hindsight of bacteriology's advent.

5. Ian F. A. Bell, *Washington Square: Styles of Money* (Woodbridge: Twayne, 1993).

6. Ibid.

7. Ibid., 43; emphasis original.

8. James, *Washington Square*, 18.

9. Bell, *Washington Square*, 24.

10. James, *Washington Square*, 3.

11. Ibid., 5.

12. Ibid., 3; 9.

13. This widely acknowledged fact can be found in many sources, including: Brodsky, *The Control of Childbirth*, 79; Bynum, *Science and the Practice of Medicine in The Nineteenth-Century*, 202; Leavitt, *Brought to Bed*, 40; Michaelson, *Childbirth in America*, 2; Rooks, *Midwifery and Childbirth in America*, 19; Wertz and Wertz, *Lying-In*, 54–65.

14. James, *Washington Square*, 4.

15. Ibid., 19.

16. Ibid., 6; emphasis mine.

17. Ibid.

18. Ibid.

19. Ibid., 6–7.

20. Ibid., 7.

21. Ibid., 4.

22. Wertz and Wertz, *Lying-In*, 55.

23. Ibid., 56.

24. Ibid., 72.

25. Phyllis L. Brodsky, *The Control of Childbirth: Women Versus Medicine Through the Ages* (Jefferson: McFarland, 2008), 79–80; Pamela Eakins, "The Medicalization of Birth," in *The American Way of Birth*, ed. Pamela S. Eakins (Philadelphia: Temple University Press, 1986), 18; Leavitt, *Brought to Bed*, 37–48; Karen L. Michaelson, *Childbirth in America: Anthropological Perspectives* (South Hadley: Bergin and Garvey, 1988), 2; Rooks, *Midwifery and Childbirth*, 15–23; Barbara Katz Rothman, *In Labor: Women and Power in the Birthplace* (New York: Norton, 1982), 50–53; Wertz and Wertz, *Lying-In*, 29–73.

26. Leavitt, *Brought to Bed*, 43.

27. Both Leavitt and Wertz and Wertz provide good summaries of the various strategies employed to this end.

28. James, *Washington Square*, 4.

29. Ibid., 5.

30. Wertz and Wertz, *Lying-In*, 64–65.

31. Brodsky, *The Control of Childbirth*, 67–75; W. F. Bynum, *Science and the Practice of Medicine*, 205–206; Nancy Schrom Dye, "The Medicalization of Birth," in *The American Way of Birth*, ed. Pamela S. Eakins (Philadelphia: Temple University Press, 1986), 36; Rothman, *In Labor*, 53; Edward Shorter, *A History of Women's Bodies* (New York: Basic Books, 1982), 103–38.

32. Brodsky, *The Control of Childbirth*, 70–71; Bynum, *Science and Medicine*, 206; Wertz and Wertz, *Lying-In*, 121.

33. Sherwin B. Nuland, "The Enigma of Semmelweis—an Interpretation," in *The Etiology, The Concept, and the Prophylaxis of Childbed Fever* (Birmingham: Classics of Medicine Library, 1981). It ought to be mentioned, as well, that in some ways, Semmelweis's work may genuinely not have seemed credible. He was, after all using innovative modes of statistical reasoning to support a brand new cosmology of disease and yet also refusing to publish his work, offering little that his colleagues around the world could use to verify his reasoning for themselves.

34. Brodsky, *The Control of Childbirth*, 72; Leavitt, *Brought to Bed*, 155–58; Wertz and Wertz, *Lying-In*, 120–24.

35. Holmes, 104.

36. Ibid., 105.

37. Ibid., 105–106.

38. Hugh L. Hodge, *On the Non-Contagious Character of Puerperal Fever* (Philadelphia: 1853), 12–13.

39. Qtd. in Nuland, "Enigma of Semmelweis," xxxv.

40. Ibid., xxxvii.

41. Ibid.

42. Ibid.

43. John Shaw, *Antiseptics in Obstetric Nursing* (London: H. K. Lewis, 1890), 1–2. Holmes also quotes this physician, Charles Meigs, in the epigraph to his famous essay.

44. Shorter, *Women's Bodies*, 104.

45. James, *Washington Square*, 6.

46. Bell, *Washington Square*, 44.

47. Ibid., 5.

48. James, *Washington Square*, 7.

49. Ibid., 45.

50. Ibid., 83.

51. Ibid.

52. Ibid., 7; 12.

53. Ibid., 84.

54. Ibid.

55. Ibid., 226; emphasis mine.

56. Ibid., 226.

57. Ibid., 144.

58. Ibid., 130.

59. Ibid., 143.

60. Ibid.

61. Ibid., 86. Catherine is of majority and could choose to marry Townsend against her father's wishes.

62. Ibid.

63. Ibid.

64. Ibid., 150.

65. Ibid.

66. Ibid., 147.

67. Ibid., 230.

68. Ibid., 231.

69. Ibid., 233.

70. Catherine does, of course, inherit and live in her father's house for the rest of her life. The domestic nature of this setting, however, further underscores her resistance to male activities and her retreat into what would have been traditionally coded as a female space while simultaneously appropriating the masculine abode of her widowed father.

71. Ibid., 225.

72. Ibid., 227.

73. Catherine plainly states her belief in these facts several times during the novel. She tells her father "I am not magnificent" in the fourth chapter, and later claims to be cowardly in a conversation with Townsend. In this same conversation, she matter-of-factly tells Townsend that there is "little . . . in me to be proud of. I am ugly and stupid." Ibid., 28; 66.

74. Ibid., 12–16.

75. Ibid., 104.

76. Ivor Grattan-Guinness, *The Norton History of the Mathematical Sciences: The Rainbow of Mathematics* (New York: Norton, 1998), 500.

77. James, *Washington Square*, 231.

78. Ibid.

79. Ibid., 243.

80. Ibid., 248.

Chapter 3. Separation and Suffocation

1. Susan Sontag, *Illness as Metaphor* (New York: McGraw-Hill, 1978), 5.

2. Ibid.

3. Katherine Ott, *Fevered Lives: Tuberculosis in American Culture since 1870* (Boston: Harvard University Press, 1996), 7.

4. I am indebted to Rupal Bhimani, MD, for these data.

5. Simon Sretzer, among others, now acknowledges that the endemicity of TB in Victorian Britain was likely only possible, in fact, because of other issues of immune suppression brought about by chronic exposure to other diseases, as well as nutritional and other environmental hazards prevalent at the time. Simon Szreter, *Health and Wealth: Studies in History and Policy* (Rochester: University of Rochester Press, 2007).

6. Georgina Feldberg, *Disease and Class: Tuberculosis and the Shaping of Modern North American Society* (New Brunswick: Rutgers University Press, 1995), 11.

7. Carolyn Day, *The Consumptive Chic: A History of Beauty, Fashion, and Disease* (New York: Bloomsbury, 2017).

8. William Dale, *A Popular, Non-Technical, Treatise on Consumption, with Remarks on Infection, Heredity, Causes, Etc.* (Harrogate: R. Ackrill, 1884), 14.

9. Katherine Byrne, *Tuberculosis and the Victorian Literary Imagination* (Cambridge: Cambridge University Press, 2013), 16.

10. Byrne similarly notes this dynamic.

11. Clark Lawlor, *Consumption and Literature: The Making of a Romantic Disease* (Basingstoke: Palgrave Macmillan, 2006), 5; Linda Bryder, *Below the Magic Mountain: A Social History of Tuberculosis in Twentieth-Century Britain* (Oxford: Clarendon Press, 1988), 1; Georgina D. Feldberg, *Disease and Class: Tuberculosis and the Shaping of Modern North American Society* (New Brunswick: Rutgers University Press, 1995), 11.

12. Rene Dubos and Jean Dubos, *The White Plague: Tuberculosis, Man, and Society* (New Brunswick: Rutgers University Press, 1987), 3.

13. Ott, *Fevered Lives*, 1.

14. Ibid.

15. Ibid., 2.

16. Ibid.

17. Byrne, *Tuberculosis*, 5; emphasis mine.

18. Ibid., 45.

19. Feldberg, *Disease and Class*, 14.

20. Qtd. in ibid., 45.

21. Ibid., 43–48.

22. Qtd. in ibid., 45.

23. Anthony Trollope, *The Ordeal of Richard Feverel* (New York: Modern Library, 1859) 178.

24. Feldberg, *Disease and Class*, 7.

25. Dubos and Dubos and Lawlor assert that one in four Victorians died of tuberculosis. Dubos and Dubos, *White Plague*, 9; Lawlor, *Consumption*, 5.

26. Charlotte Brontë, *Jane Eyre* (New York: Norton, 2000), 57.

27. Ibid., 64–65.

28. Ibid., 65; 70.

29. Ibid., 70.

30. Ibid., 69. The notion of "contagion" predates the germ theory cosmology that would later give it structure and cultural heft.

31. Ibid., 67.

32. Priscilla Wald, *Contagious: Cultures, Carriers, and the Outbreak Narrative* (Durham: Duke University Press, 2008), 2.

33. Lawlor, *Consumption*, 111; 1–2.

34. Byrne, *Tuberculosis*, 47.

35. Dubos and Dubos, *White Plague*, 9.

36. Lawlor, *Consumption*, 1–2.

37. Ibid., 10.

38. Ibid., 166.

39. Brontë, *Jane Eyre*, 68.

40. Ibid.

41. Ibid.

42. Ibid., 69.

43. Ibid., 70.

44. Ibid., 65.

45. Ibid., 68.

46. Ibid., 70.

47. Harriet Beecher Stowe, *Uncle Tom's Cabin* (New York: Norton, 1994), 258; 260.

48. Mary Armstrong, "Reading a Head: *Jane Eyre*, Phrenology, and the Homoerotics of Legibility," *Victorian Literature and Culture* 33, no. 1 (2005): 118.

49. There is one exception. Jane recalls Helen's deathbed scene when she attends Mrs. Reed at her deathbed.

50. Armstrong, "Reading a Head,"127.

51. Miss Mitford, "Female Friendship," *The Literary Panorama* (May 1813): 672.

52. "Women's Friendships," *Saturday Review*, April 1866, 497.

53. Ibid., 498.

54. Ellen Wood, *East Lynne* (Oxford: Oxford University Press, 2008), 180.

55. Ibid., 112.

56. Ibid., 114.

57. Ibid.

58. Ibid., 115.

59. Ibid., 147. Barbara and Carlyle have many conversations like this, and the subject is always their strategy to exonerate her brother, Richard, of false murder charges.

60. Ibid., 245.

61. Ibid.

62. Ibid., 256.

63. Ibid., 411.

64. Ibid., 180.

65. Ibid., 152; 77.

66. Ibid., 163.

67. Ibid., 164.

68. Ibid., 123.

69. Ibid.

70. Ibid., 167.

71. Tess Cosslett, *Woman to Woman: Female Friendships in Victorian Fiction* (Ann Arbor: University of Michigan Press, 1988).

72. Of course, Joyce is the singular exception to Isabel's world of female rivalry. The novel seems to insist that, as a servant, Joyce's friendship with Isabel does not threaten the household order. However, their friendship remains an anomaly, not only in *East Lynne*, but also in Victorian fiction more generally. *Jane Eyre* illustrates nothing if not the anxiety that servants such as governesses provoked for Victorian readers, and Isabel herself represents a threat to middle-class morality when she returns to East Lynne in the guise of a governess. That is, while the novel insists that friendships that straddle class boundaries are somehow safer than same-class friendships, the novel later negates its own assertions that there are *any* realms of safety in which a woman can place her affections.

73. Wood, *East Lynne*, 182.

74. Ibid., 9.

75. Ibid., 9. Dubos and Dubos, *White Plague*, 80.

76. "Consumption," in *Chambers's Edinburgh Journal*, Oct. 3, 1835, 282.

77. Dubos and Dubos, *White Plague*, 28–43.

78. Wood, *East Lynne*, 168.

79. Ibid., 148.

80. Ibid.

81. Ibid., 167.

82. Ibid., 94.

83. Ibid., 108.

84. Ibid., 105.

85. Cynthia Eagle Russett, *Sexual Science* (Cambridge: Harvard University Press, 1989), 68.

86. Clark Lawlor uses the term "good death" (among others) in his work *Consumption and Literature: The Making of the Romantic Disease.* Beller has also applied the same term to any romanticized female death that seeks to "ensure that the perfection exhibited by the woman in life is preserved in the moment of transition." Since this term represents a point of intersection between scholars of consumption and scholars of femininity and mortality in the Victorian era, it is particularly apt here. Anne-Marie Beller, "Suffering Angels: Death and Femininity in Ellen Wood's Fiction," *Women's Writing* 15, no. 2 (2008): 222.

87. Anne-Marie Beller, "Suffering Angels," 225.

88. Ibid., 229.

89. Wood, *East Lynne*, 618.

90. Mary Elizabeth Braddon, *John Marchmont's Legacy* (Oxford: Oxford University Press, 1999), 41; 10.

91. Ibid., 63.

92. Ibid., 64.

93. Ibid.

94. Ibid., 22.

95. Ibid., 49. Recall that Isabel is described as "almost painfully considerate of the feelings of others." Wood, *East Lynne*, 148.

96. Braddon, *John Marchmont*, 131.

97. Arundel later laments, "To think that I was so wretched a dupe! To think that my dull ears could hear that sound, and no instinct rise up in my heart to reveal the presence of my child!" Ibid., 431.

98. The differences between this viewpoint and the mid-century perspective are subtle. While mid-century discourse relied upon Darwinian notions of inheritance and contaminated bloodlines, *fin-de-siècle* perspectives specifically leaned upon a more modern understanding of a specific lack of immunity to certain microbes.

99. Karl Pearson, *Tuberculosis, Heredity, and the Environment* (1912).

100. Ibid., 46.

101. William L Russell, "Consumption: The Conditions Which Invite a Foothold of this Dread Disease," *Maine Farmer*, Feb. 3, 1897, 2.

102. Ibid.

103. Dubos and Dubos, *White Plague*, 4; Lawlor, *Consumption*, 5.

104. Beller, "Suffering Angels," 226.

105. Several scholars have noted the connection of this notion in Dixon's novel to the events leading up to the repeal of the CDA, elucidated in the previous chapter.

106. Emma Liggins, "Writing against the 'Husband-Fiend'; Syphilis and Male Sexual Vice in the New Woman Novel," *Women's Writing* 7, no. 2 (2000): 184.

107. Ella Hepworth Dixon, *The Story of a Modern Woman* (London: Broadview, 2004), 166.

108. Ibid., 167.

109. Ibid.

110. Ibid.

111. Ibid., 164.

112. Liggins, "Husband-Fiend," 184.

113. Athena Vrettos, *Somatic Fictions: Imagining Illness in Victorian Culture* (Stanford: Stanford University Press, 1995), 3.

114. Dixon, *Modern Woman,* 164.

115. Ibid.

116. Ibid., 165.

117. Ibid., 189.

118. Ibid.

Chapter 4. Tainted Love

1. Margaret Oliphant, "The Anti-Marriage League," *Blackwood's Magazine,* Jan. 1896, 135.

2. William Archer, "The Drama in the Doldrums," *Fortnightly Review,* Aug. 1892, 149.

3. Thomas Hardy, "In Tenebris II," 14.

4. Donald L. Hoffman's article "Hard(l)y Tristan" compares *Hedda Gabler* and *Jude the Obscure*, while Paul Binding's "Built to Last: Creative Connections between Ibsen and Hardy" compares *The Master Builder* with *Jude the Obscure*. Ross Shideler also devotes his book *Questioning the Father: From Darwin to Zola, Ibsen, Strindberg, and Hardy* in part to this topic.

5. James Mcarlane, ed., *The Cambridge Companion to Ibsen* (Cambridge: Cambridge University Press, 1994), xvi–xx.

6. This fact is both widely critically recognized and evident from the letters of both men; further, Archer produced many of the first definitive English translations of Ibsen's plays. Interestingly, in a January 1891 letter to his wife Emma, Hardy briefly mentions that "Gosse has been attacked in last nights [*sic*] *Pall Mall*," referring to Archer's criticism of Gosse's own translation of *Hedda Gabler* (*Letters*, 61–62).

7. Both Tess Durbeyfield and Nora Helmer from *A Doll's House,* for instance, abandon the men to whom they ostensibly rightfully "belong" in favor of their own

aims, and both Jude Fawley and Ragnar Brovik from *The Master Builder*, architects from the lower classes, struggle against rigid class structures.

8. The reaction to *Ghosts* is a critical commonplace, mentioned in virtually every text devoted to the subject.

9. Qtd. in G. B. Shaw, *Quintessence of Ibsenism* (New York: Hill and Wang, 1958), 91.

10. Timothy Carlo Matos, "Choleric Fictions: Epidemiology, Medical Authority, and *An Enemy of the People*," *Modern Drama* 51, no. 3 (2008): 353.

11. Qtd. in ibid.

12. Ibid.

13. Evert Sprinchorn, "Syphilis in Ibsen's *Ghosts*," *Ibsen Studies* 4, no. 2 (2004): 192.

14. W. H. P., "The Ibsen Bacillus," *The National Observer* Nov. 28, 1896, 41.

15. "More Morbid than Ibsen," *Saturday Review* 77, Feb. 29, 1894, 191.

16. "*Tess of the D'Urbervilles*," *Novel Review*, March 1892, 285.

17. Qtd. in Helmut E. Gerber and W. Eugene Davis, *Thomas Hardy: An Annotated Bibliography of Writings about Him* (De Kalb: Northern Illinois University Press, 1973), 68.

18. Ibid., 31.

19. Ibid., 75.

20. Ibid., 68.

21. Ibid., 19.

22. Francis W. Newman, *The Cure of the Great Social Evil, with Special Reference to Recent Laws Delusively Called Contagious Diseases' Acts* (London: Trubner, 1869), 6. Judith R. Walkowitz, *Prostitution and Victorian Society: Women, Class, and the State* (Cambridge: Cambridge University Press, 1980), 76.

23. Newman, *Cure of the Great Social Evil*, 6.

24. Sprinchorn, "Syphilis," 192. For more information about [the] European legislation that inspired the CDA, see *History of Sexuality in Europe*, ed. Anna Clark.

25. Mary Spongberg, *Feminizing Venereal Disease: The Body of the Prostitute in Nineteenth-Century Medical Discourse* (New York: NYU Press, 1997), 7; 143; Walkowitz, *Prostitution*, 70.

26. Spongberg, *Feminizing Venereal Disease*, 6.

27. *Sanitary Perspective* 2.

28. This is the debate over whether the laws were efficacious at all.

29. That is, whether good or bad.

30. Christopher Bulteel, *Contagious Disease Acts Considered in their Moral, Social, and Sanitary Aspects* (London: Robert Hardwicke, 1870).

31. Newman, *Cure of the Great Social Evil*, 11.

32. *Licencing Prostitution* (London: Unwin Bros., 1869), 17; emphasis original.

33. *The Remedy Worse than the Disease* (London: 1869), 7; emphasis original.

34. Elizabeth Garrett, *An Enquiry into the Character of the Contagious Disease Acts* (London: 1870), 9.

35. *The Contagious Diseases Acts: Or, a Few Suggestions for Controlling Men as Well as Women* (London: 1873), 4–5.

36. C. W. Shirley Deakin, *The Contagious Diseases Acts* (London: University College Medical Society, 1872), 2.

37. Spongberg, *Feminizing Venereal Disease*, 9.

38. Deakin, *Contagious Diseases Acts*, 4.

39. Newman, *Cure of the Great Social Evil*, 23.

40. *Licencing Prostitution*, 19; emphasis original.

41. *Remedy Worse than the Disease*, 4; emphasis original.

42. Newman, *Cure of the Great Social Evil*, 12–13; emphasis original.

43. Ibid.

44. Ibid., 6.

45. Garrett, *An Enquiry*, 1; emphasis mine.

46. William Acton, *The Contagious Disease Acts: Shall the Contagious Disease Acts Be Applied to the Civil Population?* (London: John Churchill & Sons, 1870); 12, emphasis mine.

47. Deakin, *Contagious Diseases Acts*, 15–16. Deakin quotes these proofs as being six in number:

1. The woman's own personal admission.

2. Residence in a brothel.

3. Habitual association with prostitutes.

4. Habitually frequenting the haunts of prostitution.

5. Soliciting publicly in the streets.

6. Being informed against by men in the army and navy as having diseased them. (16)

48. Newman, *Cure of the Great Social Evil*, 5.

49. Charles Bell Taylor, *Observations on the Contagious Disease Acts* (Nottingham: 1869), 7.

50. Deakin, *Contagious Diseases Act*, 22.

51. Garrett, *An Enquiry*, 9.

52. Deakin, *Contagious Diseases Acts*, 20.

53. Ibid., 26.

54. Bulteel, *Contagious Disease Acts Considered*.

55. Newman, *Cure of the Great Social Evil*, 12.

56. Ibid.

57. Ibid., 152.

58. Virtually every study of the social history of syphilis deals with the contemporary dilemma of whether or not syphilitics ought to marry. Mary Spongberg, Barbara Fass Leavy, Emma Liggins, and Andrew Smith discuss this issue at length. Nearly all of these studies cite Fournier as a singular advocate for women. Barbara Fass Leavy, *To Blight with Plague* (New York: NYU Press, 1992); Emma Liggins, "Writing against the 'Husband-Fiend'; Syphilis and Male Sexual Vice in the New Woman Novel," *Women's Writing* 7, no. 2 (2000); Andrew Smith, *Victorian Demons: Medicine, Masculinity, and the Gothic at the* fin-de-siècle (Manchester: Manchester University Press, 2004).

59. Qtd. in Spongberg, *Feminizing Venereal Disease*, 149; emphasis original.

60. Qtd. in ibid., 154. Andrew Smith notes that, while Hutchison dedicated his 1887 text *Syphilis* to Fournier, he nevertheless diverged from Fournier, who insisted that careless men risked great harm to their wives in adopting "the recurring narrative . . . that men contract the disease in a way which suggests . . . that they are innocent victims." Smith, *Victorian Demons,* 108.

61. Smith, *Victorian Demons,* 108–109.

62. Ibid., 109.

63. Qtd. in Smith, *Victorian Demons,* 109.

64. Smith, *Victorian Demons,* 115.

65. Ibid.

66. Henrik Ibsen, *Ghosts,* trans. James McFarlane (Oxford: Oxford University Press, 1994), 114.

67. Ibid., 118. In fact, Ibsen himself wrote that "after Nora, Mrs. Alving had to come." Qtd. in Joan Templeton, "Advocacy and Ambivalence in Ibsen's Drama," *Ibsen Studies* 7, no. 1 (2007): 43–60.

68. Ibsen, *Ghosts,* 118.

69. Ibid., 117.

70. Ibid., 125.

71. Ibid., 119.

72. Ibid.

73. Ibid., 104.

74. Ross Shideler, *Questioning the Father: From Darwin to Zola, Ibsen, Strindberg, and Hardy* (Stanford: Stanford University Press, 1999), 62–63.

75. Ibsen, *Ghosts,* 138.

76. Ibid., 124.

77. Ibid., 139.

78. Ibid., 138.

79. Ibid., 125; 112; emphasis mine.

80. Ibid., 161. Ibsen's personal knowledge of syphilis is highlighted in these turns of phrase. His good friend Georg Brandes had fallen in love with a married woman whose husband had syphilis. In 1875, Ibsen commiserated with Brandes's and

his lover's miserable situation by writing a poem discussing "the ship of civilization" that "carries 'a corpse in the cargo.'" Sprinchorn, "Syphilis," 194. The meticulous research that went into *Ghosts* is also evident here, as "softening of the brain" is precisely the term Fournier used. Sprinchorn, "Syphilis," 195.

81. Ibsen, *Ghosts,* 160.

82. A. F. Machiraju, "Ideals and Victims: Ibsen's Concerns in *Ghosts* and *The Wild Duck,*" *Modern Language Review* 87, no. 1 (1992): 139.

83. Ibid.

84. Ibsen, *Ghosts,* 126; emphasis original.

85. Ibid., 153.

86. Ibid., 159.

87. Ibid., 163.

88. Ibid., 164.

89. Thomas Hardy, *The Woodlanders* (Oxford: Oxford University Press, 1985), 121.

90. Ibid.

91. Ibid., 231.

92. Ibid., 227.

93. Ibid.

94. Ibid., 225.

95. Ibid.

96. Ibid., 228.

97. Ibid., 207.

98. Ibid., 224.

99. Ibid.

100. Ibid., 221.

101. Ibid., 226.

102. Ibid., 227.

103. Ibid., 231.

104. Ibid.; emphasis mine.

105. Ibid., 232.

106. Ibid., 233; emphasis original.

107. Although Hardy does not specify Giles's illness (Edred surmises it may be typhoid fever, though I would argue it manifests more like tuberculosis), it is clear that he does not have a traditional STD such as syphilis or gonorrhea. However, because Grace contracts his illness *via sexual contact* in the act of kissing his lips, I argue that Hardy renders Grace's illness a sexually transmitted disease in the most denotative of meanings. Perhaps by sidestepping the obviously sexual undertones of *Ghosts, Tess of the D'Urbervilles,* and *Jude the Obscure,* Hardy hoped to create a text whose social meaning was less initially reviled by scandalized critics.

108. Ibid., 236.

109. Ibid., 228.

110. Ibid., 226; 229–30.

111. Indeed, to this end, Joanna Devereux notes that *The Woodlanders* "most clearly anticipates the attack on patriarchal values in *Tess of the D'Urbervilles* and *Jude the Obscure*." Joanna Devereux, *Patriarchy and its Discontents: Sexualized Politics in Selected Novels and Stories of Thomas Hardy* (New York: Routledge, 2003), 71. In her chapter on *The Woodlanders,* Devereux also notes the ways in which Giles's function as "the epitome of masculine virtue" results in his ceasing to signify as a male at all in the text through the "self-denial of passion" mandated by Victorian gender norms; thus, he ultimately serves to highlight "the inordinately high price to be paid for gentlemanliness in the later decades of the century." Devereux, *Patriarchy*, 69–74.

112. Hardy, *The Woodlanders*, 235.

113. Ibid., 247; 241.

114. Phillotson's fate in *Jude the Obscure* is a good representative example of the fates awaiting forgiving husbands.

115. Ibid., 241.

116. Melbury throws Edred off a horse and leaves him for dead, resulting in Edred's resolution to forever shun him.

117. Ibid., 222.

118. Ibid., 240–41.

119. Ibid.

120. Ibid., 253.

121. Ibid., 250.

122. Ibid., 256.

123. Ibid., 248.

124. Thomas Hardy, *Jude the Obscure* (New York: Barnes and Noble, 2003), 172; emphasis mine.

125. Ibid., 133.

126. Ibid., 362.

127. Ibid., 282.

128. Ibid., 282; 303; 287.

129. *A Treatise on Syphilis in New-Born Children*, 86.

130. Alfred Fournier, *Syphilis and Marriage* (New York: D. Appleton, 1882), 55.

131. Edward Ellis, *Diseases of Childhood* (New York: William Wood, 1879), 22.

132. Wellcome Collection, taken from "A nine week old baby girl with diseased skin on her face, arms and body, displaying symptoms of hereditary syphilis." Watercolour by C. D'Alton, 1856 and Franz Mracek, *Atlas of Syphilis and the Venereal Diseases* (London: Rebman, 1898), respectively.

133. Hardy, *Jude*, 286; 345.

134. Elaine Showalter has argued for Little Father Time as suffering from congenital syphilis in her book *Sex, Politics, and Science in the Nineteenth-Century Novel.*

135. Ibid., 348.

136. Ibid., 330.

137. Ibid., 285.

138. Ibid., 317; 295.

139. Ibid., 335.

140. Ibid., 332.

141. Ibid., 314.

142. Ibid., 282.

143. Ibid., 345.

144. Ibid. Talia Schaffer, *The Forgotten Female Aesthetes: Literary Culture in Late-Victorian England* (Charlottesville: University of Virginia Press, 2000), 238. Sally Shuttleworth, "The Psychology of Childhood in Victorian Literature and Medicine," in *Literature, Science, Psychoanalysis, 1830–1970,* ed. Gillian Beer, Helen Small, and Trudi Tate (Oxford: Oxford University Press, 2003), 98.

145. Hardy, *Jude*, 293.

146. Ibid., 340.

147. Ibid., 281.

148. Ibid., 344–45.

149. Ibid., 345.

150. Ibid., 351.

151. Ibid., 280.

152. Ibid., 281.

153. Ibid., 396.

154. Ibid., 398–99.

155. Ibid., 399.

156. Ibid., 378.

157. Ibid., 399.

158. Ibid., 397–99.

159. Ibid., 362.

160. Ibid., 400.

161. Ibid., 413.

Chapter 5. Humanity's Waste

1. This should not, of course, be conflated with Catherine Sloper's radical isolation-as-resistance in *Washington Square*. This will become clear, as the isolationist efforts I track in this chapter have to do with personal beliefs (on the part of the protagonists) in moral superiority as justification for moral separatism.

2. William A. Davis Jr., "Reading Failure In(to) *Jude The Obscure*: Hardy's Sue Bridehead and Lady Jeune's 'New Woman' Essays 1885–1900," *Victorian Literature and Culture* 26, no. 1 (1998): 53.

3. Ibid., 54.

4. British Library Collections, https://www.bl.uk/collection-items/the-woman-who-did-a-novel.

5. Grant Allen, *The Woman Who Did*, 44.

6. Ibid., 158.

7. Ibid., 46–48.

8. Ibid., Appendix 4, 213.

9. Ibid., 217.

10. Ibid., 220.

11. Ibid.; emphasis mine.

12. Ibid., 224.

13. Ibid., 159.

14. Ibid., 90.

15. Ibid., 119.

16. Ibid., 122.

17. Ibid., 101.

18. Ibid., 131.

19. Ibid.

20. Ibid., 84.

21. Mary Douglas, *Purity and Danger* (New York: Routledge, 1966 /2002), 44.

22. Allen, *The Woman Who Did*, 179.

23. Ibid., 143.

24. *How to Avoid Typhoid and Other Allied Diseases*, 1.

25. Allen, *The Woman Who Did*, 110.

26. Ibid., 104; emphasis mine.

27. Ibid., 109–12.

28. Ibid., 114.

29. Ibid.

30. Arthur Henry Downes, *How To Avoid Typhoid Fever* (London: 1876), 1.

31. Baldwin Latham, *The Utilisation of Sewage* (London: E and F. N., 1867), b.

32. Hamlin, 198.

33. Latham, *The Utilisation of Sewage*, 21.

34. *Bacteriology of Sewage*, 179.

35. Thomas Spencer, *On the Quality of the New River Company's Water* (London: Gilbert and Rivington, 1855), 31.

36. *Bacterial Treatment of Sewage*, 185.

37. Ibid.

38. E. Bailey-Denton, *Sewage Purification Brought Up to Date* (New York: Spon and Chamberlain, 1896), 4.

39. *Bacterial Treatment of Sewage*, 189–97.

40. *How to Make a House Sanitary*, 5.

41. G. V. Poore, *Dry Methods of Sanitation* (London: Edward Stanford, 1894), 1.

42. *How to Make a House Sanitary.*

43. Ibid.

44. Downes, *How To Avoid Typhoid Fever,* 1.

45. *How to Make a House Sanitary,* 17.

46. Ibid., 18–20.

47. Poore, *Dry Methods,* 4.

48. Downes, *How to Avoid Typhoid Fever,* 22.

49. P. Hinckes Bird. *Hints on Drains, Traps, Closets, Sewer Gas, and Sewage Disposal* (Blackpool: Gazette), 28. Wellcome Online Collections.

50. Michelle Allen, "From Cesspool to Sewer: Sanitary Reform and the Rhetoric of Resistance, 1848–1880," *Victorian Literature and Culture* 30, no. 2 (2002): 393.

51. Ibid., 391.

52. Qtd above.

53. "New Theatrical Bills," *New York Times* April 9, 1895.

54. "Review of 'An Enemy of the People,'" *The Referee,* July 22, 1894.

55. Katherine E. Kelley, "Pandemic Performance and Outbreak of Modernism," *South Central Review* 25, no. 1 (2008): 23.

56. Thomas F. Van Laan, "Generic Complexity in Ibsen's 'An Enemy of the People,'" *Comparative Drama* 20, no. 2 (1986): 96.

57. Merete Morken Andersen, "The Artist as an Enemy of the People: Ibsen in the Perspective of Role Theory," in *Proceedings of the 2006 International Ibsen Conference,* 5.

58. Henrik Ibsen, *An Enemy of the People,* trans. James McFarlane (Oxford: Oxford University Press, 1988), 106.

59. Magne Nylenna. "Dr. Stockmann og Dr. Snow—to Samfunnsmedisinske Helter," *Tidsskriftet: Den Norske Legeforening,* Dec. 18 2003. All translations, unless otherwise noted, are my own.

60. Ibid.

61. P. Vinten-Johansen, "Dr. Stockmann and Dr. Snow," *Tidsskriftet: Den Norske Legeforening,* Aug. 1 2004.

62. Stephen Wallace, "Governing Humanity," *Journal for Medical Humanities* 29 (2008): 29–31.

63. Van Laan, "Generic Complexity," 96. It is clear from this excerpt that Van Laan complicates this reading, but he no more reads Stockmann as an enemy than as a hero. Instead, he argues that Ibsen is playing with several dramatic types and blending them as a sort of theatrical thought experiment.

64. Ibsen, *Enemy of the People,* 73.

65. Ibid.

66. Ibid., 76.

67. Ibid.

68. Ibid., 77.

69. Ibid.

70. Ibid.

71. Ibid., 78.

72. Ibid., 74.

73. Ibid.

74. Ibid., 79.

75. Ibid., 80.

76. Ibid., 82.

77. Ibid., 87.

78. Thomas Adler, "Conscience and Community in *An Enemy of the People* and *The Crucible,*" in *The Cambridge Companion to Arthur Miller* (Cambridge: Cambridge University Press, 1997), 87.

79. This can be found in nearly any source that talks about the play, but some examples include Merete Morken Anderson, Stephen Wallace, and Hub Zwart, among others.

80. Paul Lindholdt, "Greening the Dramatic Canon: Henrik Ibsen's 'An Enemy of the People,'" *Interdisciplinary Literary Studies* 3, no. 1 (2001): 56.

81. "Ibsen at Lyceum Friday," *Cornell Daily Sun*, March 6, 1909, 4.

82. Ibid.

83. Ibid.

84. "Ibsen in Paris," *The Times*, Nov. 13, 1893; 5, emphasis mine.

85. The Referee.

86. "Ibsen Play Superbly Rendered," *Ithaca Daily News*, March 1909.

87. Theater Season Program, "Nationaltheatrets repertoire 1ste season 1899–1900."

88. L. B. "Nationaltheatret." Program Notes.

89. Ibsen, *Enemy of the People*, 17.

90. Ibid., 34.

91. Ibid., 17.

92. Ibid., 9; 39.

93. Hub Zwart, "Environmental Pollution and Professional Responsibility: Ibsen's *A Public Enemy* as a Seminar on Science Communication and Ethics," *Environmental Values* 13 (2004): 364.

94. Ibsen, *Enemy of the People*, 18.

95. Ibid., 19.

96. Hub Zwart has similarly noted that Doctor Stockmann "is far from being Koch's equal," and has also observed that Stockmann's work "remained heavily dependent on the tools and expertise of others." However, he takes at face value that Stockmann has truly found something dangerous in the town's water—and in any event, Zwart, while providing important parallels among Stockmann, Koch, and Pasteur, relegates Stockmann's mistake to that of "his unwise decision to change genres and to leap from science to political philosophy without preparing himself properly." Zwart, "Professional Responsibility," 368. Frederik Engelstad has written one of the only other discussions of Stockmann as compared to contemporary scientists, but also takes a philosophical approach in his very interesting article. He

likens Stockmann to Semmelweis and argues that Stockmann's downfall is the result of his refusal to accept that "science is nothing but social conventions." "Knowledge and Society. Holberg, Ibsen, and Bjørneboe," *Norwegian Literature* 1995 (Special issue of *The Norseman* 4/5 1995): 17–25; translation mine.

97. Ibsen, *Enemy of the People*, 18.

98. *Bacteriology of Sewage*, 179.

99. Ibid., 180.

100. Ibid., 183.

101. Edvard Brandes, "Henrik Ibsen: 'En Folkefiende,'" *Ude og Hjemme*, March 11, 1883.

102. Ibid.

103. Arthur Miller, "A Letter from Arthur Miller," in *An Enemy of the People* Theater program, Feb. 1971.

104. Qtd in Van Laan, "Generic Complexity," 96.

105. Lindholdt, "Greening the Dramatic Canon," 54.

106. Arno K. Lepke, "Who Is Doctor Stockmann?" *Scandinavian Studies* 32, no. 2 (1960): 59.

107. Ibid.

108. Ibid.

109. Zwart, "Professional Responsibility," 362.

110. "Ibsen Play Superbly Rendered."

111. Ibid. Ibsen was trained as a pharmacist, and hence often called Dr. Ibsen. It is this to which the author refers when he says "no one knows better than Ibsen" what some doctors would recommend.

112. Another relevant change, though not relevant for discussion here, is his substitution of Florence for Flora in the later manuscript, which may have been made to appease his second wife, Florence Dugdale Hardy.

113. Thomas Hardy, *The Well-Beloved* (New York: Wordsworth Classics, 2000), 3.

114. Ibid.

115. *How to Make a House Sanitary*, 17.

116. Poore, *Dry Methods*, 13.

117. Advertisement, "Macfarlane's Pipes," in John Hart, *Hints to Plumbers on Joint Wiping, Pipe Bending, and Lead Burning* (London: Smith and Greenwood, 1896), 315; Wellcome Online Collections.

118. Hardy, *The Well-Beloved*, 158.

Conclusion

1. I am indebted to Claire Hooker's considerations of disease, proposed for *Endemic: Essays in Contagion Theory*, ed. Kari Nixon and Lorenzo Servitje (Palgrave Macmillan, forthcoming), for these revisionist considerations of epidemics.

2. See, for instance, "Sierra Leone Loses its 10th Doctor to Ebola Outbreak," *CBSNews.com*, Dec. 7, 2014.

3. Images taken by the author.

4. "Public Disinfectors," in John Thomson and Adolphe Smith, *Victorian London Street Life in Historic Photographs* (London: Sampson, Low, 1877).

5. Grant Allen, *The Woman Who Did* (Boston: Roberts Brothers, 1895), 178.

6. Julia Kristeva, *Powers of Horror: An Essay on Abjection* (New York: Columbia University Press, 1982), 4.

7. Ibid., 1–2.

8. Ibid.

9. Anne Finger, *Elegy for a Disease: A Personal and Cultural History of Polio* (New York: St. Martins, 2006), 19–20.

10. Allen, *The Woman Who Did*, 137.

11. Ibid., 155.

12. Ibid.

13. "The Battle of the Bacilli," *The Outlook*, Dec. 30, 1899, 713.

14. Sarah Kurchak, "I'm Autistic, and Believe Me, It's a Lot Better than Measles," *Archipelago*; medium.com.

Works Cited

Acton, William. *The Contagious Disease Acts: Shall the Contagious Disease Acts be Applied to the Civil population?* London: John Churchill and Sons, 1870.

Adler, Thomas. "Conscience and Community in *An Enemy of the People* and *The Crucible*." In *The Cambridge Companion to Arthur Miller*, 87. Cambridge: Cambridge University Press, 1997.

Agamben, Giorgio. *Homo Sacer: Sovereign Power and Bare Life*. Stanford: Stanford University Press, 1995.

Allen, Grant. *The Woman Who Did*. Boston: Roberts Brothers, 1895.

Allen, Michelle. "From Cesspool to Sewer: Sanitary Reform and the Rhetoric of Resistance, 1848–1880." *Victorian Literature and Culture* 30, no. 2 (2002): 393.

Altick, Richard D. *Victorian People and Ideas: A Companion for the Modern Reader of Victorian Literature*. New York: Norton, 1974.

Andersen, Merete Morken. "The Artist as an Enemy of the People: Ibsen in the Perspective of Role Theory." Proceedings of the 2006 International Ibsen Conference, 5.

Anderson, Benedict. *Imagined Communities* London: Verso, 1983.

"Another Book on Bacteriology." *The Saturday Review*, August 1, 1891.

Armstrong, Mary. "Reading a Head: 'Jane Eyre,' Phrenology, and the Homoerotics of Legibility." *Victorian Literature and Culture* 33, no. 1 (2005): 107–32.

Armstrong, Nancy, and Leonard Tennenhouse. "Sovereignty and the Form of Formlessness." *Differences: A Journal of Feminist Cultural Studies* 20, no. 2–3 (2009): 148–78.

Archer, William. "The Drama in the Doldrums." *Fortnightly Review*, August 1892.

Arnold, Matthew. "Stanzas from the Grand Chartreuse."

Bailes, Melissa. "The Psychologization of Geological Catastrophe in Mary Shelley's *The Last Man*." *ELH* 82 (2015): 671–99.

Bailey-Denton, E. *Sewage Purification Brought up to Date*. New York: Spon and Chamberlain, 1896.

Bailin, Miriam. *The Sickroom in Victorian Fiction: The Art of Being Ill*. Cambridge: Cambridge University Press, 1994.

Baker, Brian. "Science and Literature in the Twentieth Century: From Entropy to Chaos." In *Literature and Science: Social Impact and Interaction*, edited by John H. Cartwright and Brian Baker, 243–64. Santa Barbara: ABC-CLIO, 2005.

Barnes, David. *The Great Stink of Paris and the Nineteenth-Century Struggle against Filth and Germs*. Baltimore: Johns Hopkins University Press, 2006.

"The Battle of the Bacilli." *The Outlook*, December 30, 1899.

Beaumont, Matthew. "Beginnings, Endings, Births, Deaths: Sterne, Dickens, and *Bleak House*." *Textual Practice* 26, no. 5 (2012): 807–27.

Bell, Ian A. *Defoe's Fiction*. London: Croom Helm, 1985.

———. *Washington Square: Styles of Money*. Woodbridge: Twayne, 1993.

Beller, Anne-Marie. "Suffering Angels: Death and Femininity in Ellen Wood's Fiction." *Women's Writing* 15, no. 2 (2008): 219–31.

Alan Bewell, *Romanticism and Colonial Disease*. Baltimore: Johns Hopkins University Press, 1999.

Binding, Paul. "Built to Last: Creative Connections between Ibsen and Hardy." *Times Literary Supplement*, August 4, 2006.

Bissell, Helen W. "Health, Beauty, and the Toilet." *Bow Bells*, August 19, 1892.

Blackmar, Betsy. "Rewalking the 'Walking City': Housing and Property Relations in New York City, 1780–1840." In *Material Life in America, 1600–1860*, edited by Robert Blair St. George, 371–84. Boston: Northeastern University Press, 1988.

Bochner, Salomon. *The Role of Mathematics in the Rise of Science*. Princeton: Princeton University Press, 1966.

Boumelha, Penny. *Thomas Hardy and Women: Sexual Ideology and Narrative Form*. Sussex: Harvester Press, 1982.

Braddon, Mary Elizabeth. *John Marchmont's Legacy*. Oxford: Oxford University Press, 1999.

Brandes, Edvard. "Henrik Ibsen: 'En Folkefiende.'" *Ude og Hjemme*, March 11, 1883.

British Library Collections. https://www.bl.uk/collection-items/the-woman-who-did-a-novel.

Brodsky, Phyllis L. *The Control of Childbirth: Women versus Medicine through the Ages*. Jefferson: McFarland, 2008.

Brodsley, Laurel. "Defoe's *The Journal of the Plague Year*: A Model for Stories of Plagues." In *AIDS: The Literary Response*, edited by Emmanuel S. Nelson, 11–22. New York: Twayne, 1992.

"Brompton Consumption Hospital." *The Sunday at Home*, June 28, 1862.

Brontë, Charlotte. *Jane Eyre*. New York: Norton, 2000.

Bryder, Linda. *Below the Magic Mountain: A Social History of Tuberculosis in Twentieth-Century Britain*. 1988.

Bulteel, Christopher. *Contagious Disease Acts Considered in their Moral, Social, and Sanitary Aspects*. London: Robert Hardwicke, 1870.

Bynum, W. F. *Science and the Practice of Medicine in the Nineteenth Century.* Cambridge: Cambridge University Press, 1994.

Byrne, Katherine. *Tuberculosis and the Victorian Literary Imagination.* Cambridge: Cambridge University Press, 2013.

"Carbolic Smoke Ball." *Tinsleys' Magazine,* July 1889.

"Carbolic Smoke Ball," *Strand Magazine,* January 1892, 20.

Carpenter, W. B. "The Germ-Theory of Zymotic Diseases: Considered from the Natural History Point of View." *The Nineteenth-Century: A Monthly Review,* February 1884.

Cartwright, John H. "Those Dreadful Hammers: Geology and Evolution in Nineteenth-Century Literature." In *Literature and Science: Social Impact and Interaction,* edited by John H. Cartwright and Brian Baker, 171–98. Santa Barbara: ABC-CLIO, 2005.

Chapple, J. A. V. *Science and Literature in the Nineteenth Century.* Hampshire: Macmillan, 1986.

Christensen, Allan Conrad. *Nineteenth-Century Narratives of Contagion: "Our Feverish Contact."* London: Routledge, 2005.

Clark, Anna, ed. *History of Sexuality in Europe.* New York: Routledge, 2011.

"Clarke's Blood Mixture." *The Gentleman's Magazine,* December 1896.

"Consumption." *Chambers's Edinburgh Journal,* October 3, 1835.

The Contagious Diseases Acts: Or, a few suggestions for Controlling men as well as women. London: 1873.

Cooke, Jennifer. "Writing Plague: Transforming Narrative, Witnessing, and History." In *The Tapestry of Health, Illness, and Disease,* edited by Peter L. Twohig and Vera Kalitzkus, 21–42. Amsterdam: Rodopi, 2008.

Cosslett, Tess. *Woman to Woman: Female Friendships in Victorian Fiction.* Ann Arbor: University of Michigan Press, 1988.

"The Cure of Consumption: By One Who Has Been Cured." *Pall Mall,* June 1903.

Cvetkovich, Ann. *Mixed Feelings: Feminism, Mass Culture, and Victorian Sensationalism.* New Brunswick: Rutgers University Press, 1992.

Dale, William. *A Popular, Non-Technical, Treatise on Consumption, with Remarks on Infection, Heredity, Causes, etc.* Harrogate: R. Ackrill, 1884.

Daleski, H. M. *Thomas Hardy and Paradoxes of Love.* Columbia: Missouri University Press, 1997.

Dalrymple, Theodore. "Unsyphilised Behaviour." *British Medical Journal,* August 21, 2010.

Davis, William A. Jr. "Reading Failure In(to) *Jude The Obscure:* Hardy's Sue Bridehead and Lady Jeune's 'New Woman' Essays 1885–1900." *Victorian Literature and Culture* 26 no. 1 (1998): 53–70.

Day, Carolyn *The Consumptive Chic: A History of Beauty, Fashion, and Disease.* New York: Bloomsbury, 2017.

Defoe, Daniel. *Compleat English Tradesman*. London: Charles Rivington, 1727.

———. *Due Preparations for the Plague, As for Soul as Body*. London: J. M. Dent, 1895.

———. *Journal of the Plague Year*. Oxford: Oxford University Press, 1998.

———. *Review*. New York: Columbia University Press, 1938.

DeGabriele, Peter. "Intimacy, Survival, and Resistance: Daniel Defoe's *A Journal of the Plague Year*." *ELH* 77, no. 1 (2010): 1–23.

Devereux, Joanna. *Patriarchy and Its Discontents: Sexual Politics in Selected Novels and Stories of Thomas Hardy*. New York: Routledge, 2003.

DeWitt, Anne. " 'The Actual Sky is a Horror': Thomas Hardy and the Arnoldian Conception of Science." *Nineteenth-Century Literature* 61, no. 4 (2007): 479–506.

Dickens, Charles. "Working Plans" for *Bleak House*. New York: Norton, 1977.

Dijkstra, Bram. *Defoe and Economics: The Fortunes of Roxana in the History of Interpretation*. New York: St. Martin's, 1987.

Dixon, Ella Hepworth. *The Story of a Modern Woman*. London: Broadview, 2004.

Douglas, Mary. *Purity and Danger*. New York: Routledge, 1966.

Douglass, William. *A Dissertation Concerning Inoculation of the Small-Pox*. Boston: Henchman, 1730.

Downes, Arthur Henry. *How To Avoid Typhoid Fever*. London: 1876.

Dubos, Rene, and Jean Dubos. *The White Plague: Tuberculosis, Man, and Society*. New Brunswick: Rutgers University Press, 1987.

Durbach, Nadja. *Bodily Matters*. Durham: Duke University Press, 2006.

Dutta, Shanta. *Ambivalence in Hardy: A Study of his Attitude to Women*. Basingstoke: Palgrave, 2000.

Dye, Nancy Schrom. "The Medicalization of Birth." In *The American Way of Birth*, edited by Pamela S. Eakins, 21–46. Philadelphia: Temple University Press, 1986.

Eakins, Pamela S. "The Medicalization of Birth." In *The American Way of Birth*, edited by. Pamela S. Eakins, 17–20. Philadelphia: Temple University Press, 1986.

Ellison, Katherine E. *Fatal News: Reading and Information Overload in Early Eighteenth-Century Literature*. New York: Routledge, 2006.

"Enamel soil pipe" (Advertisement). In *Lectures on Sanitary Plumbing*. London: Haldane, 1891–92.

Engelstad, Frederik. "Vitenskap og samfunn hos Holberg, Ibsen, og Bjørneboe." In *Litteratur, forskning, og etikk* De Nasjonale Forskningsetiske komiteer: Oslo: 1996.

Eno's Fruit Salt. *Longman's Magazine*, November 1897.

Feldberg, Georgina. *Disease and Class: Tuberculosis and the Shaping of Modern North American* Society. New Brunswick: Rutgers University Press, 1995.

Fincham, Tony. *Hardy the Physician: Medical Aspects of the Wessex Tradition*. Basingstoke: Palgrave, 2008.

Fournier, Alfred. *Syphilis and Marriage*, New York: D. Appleton, 1882.

Freedman, Morris. *The Moral Impulse: Modern Drama from Ibsen to the Present.* Carbondale: Southern Illinois University Press, 1967.

Fyfe, Aiyleen, and Bernard Lightman, eds. *Science in the Marketplace: Nineteenth-Century Sites and Experiences.* Chicago: University of Chicago Press, 2007.

Garrett, Elizabeth. *An Enquiry into the Character of the Contagious Disease Acts.* London: 1870.

Gerber, Helmut E., and W. Eugene Davis. *Thomas Hardy: An Annotated Bibliography of Writings about Him.* De Kalb: Northern Illinois University Press, 1973.

"The Germ Theory Again." *Chambers's Magazine*, November 1897.

" 'Ghosts' A Triumph for Mrs. Shaw." *The Evening World*, January 29, 1903.

Gossin, Pamela. *Thomas Hardy's Novel Universe: Astronomy, Cosmology, and Gender in the Post-Darwinian World.* Aldershot: Ashgate, 2007.

Grattan-Guinness, Ivor. *The Norton History of the Mathematical Sciences: The Rainbow of Mathematics.* New York: Norton, 1998.

Hardy, Thomas. *A Pair of Blue Eyes.* Hertfordshire: Wordsworth Classics, 1995.

———. "In Tenebris II."

———. *Jude the Obscure.* New York: Barnes and Noble, 2003.

———. *Life and Art.* New York: Haskell House, 1966.

———. *Literary Notebooks,* edited by Lennart A. Björk. Vol. 2. New York: New York University Press, 1985.

———. *'Poetical Matter' Notebook,* edited by Pamela Dalziel and Michael Millgate. Oxford: Oxford University Press, 2009.

———. *Two on a Tower.* New York: Penguin, 1999.

———. *Selected Letters.* Edited by Michael Millgate. Oxford: Clarendon, 1990.

———. *The Well-Beloved.* New York: Wordsworth Classics.

———. *The Woodlanders.* Oxford: Oxford University Press, 1985.

Harris, Jonathan Gil. *Foreign Bodies and the Body Politic: Discourses of Social Pathology in Early Modern England.* Cambridge: Cambridge University Press, 1998.

Healy, Margaret. "Defoe's *Journal* and the English Plague Writing Tradition." *Literature and Medicine* 22, no. 1 (2003): 25–44.

Hodge, Hugh L. *On the Non-Contagious Character of Pueperal Fever.* Philadelphia: T. K. and P. G. Collins, 1852.

Hoffman, Donald L. "Hard(l)y Tristan." In *On Arthurian Women: Essays in Memory of Maureen Fries,* edited by Bonnie Wheeler and Fiona Tolhurst, 271–82. Dallas: Scriptorium, 2001.

Holmes, Oliver Wendell. "The Contagiousness of Pueperal Fever." 1843.

How to Make a House Sanitary.

"Ibsen at lyceum Friday." *Cornell Daily Sun*, March 6, 1909.

Ibsen, Henrik. *A Doll's House.* Translated by James McFarlane. Oxford: Oxford University Press, 1961.

———. *Ghosts.* Translated by James McFarlane. Oxford: Oxford University Press, 1961.

———. *An Enemy of the People*. Translated by James McFarlane. Oxford: Oxford University Press, 1988.

———. *Letters and Speeches*. Edited by Evert Sprinchorn. New York: Hill and Wang, 1964.

"Ibsen in Paris," *The Times*, November 13, 1893.

"Ibsen Play Superbly Rendered." *Ithaca Daily News*, March 1909.

Izal Powder. *Strand Magazine,* January 1893.

James, Henry. *The Wings of the Dove*. New York: Penguin, 1986.

———. *Washington Square*. New York: The Modern Library, 2002.

Joyce, James. *The Critical Writings*. Edited by Ellsworth Mason and Richard Ellmann. New York: Viking, 1959.

Juengel, Scott J. "Writing Decomposition: Defoe and the Corpse." *The Journal of Narrative Technique* 25, no. 2 (1995): 139–53.

Keats, John. "When I Have Fears."

Kelley, Katherine E. "Pandemic Performance and Outbreak of Modernism." *South Central Review* 25, no. 1 (2008): 23.

Kohn, George Childs, ed. *Encyclopedia of Plague and Pestilence: From Ancient Times to the Present*. 3rd ed. New York: Facts on File, 2008.

Kristeva, Julia. *Powers of Horror: An Essay on Abjection*. New York: Columbia University Press, 1982.

Kuhn, Thomas. *The Structure of Scientific Revolutions*. Chicago: University of Chicago Press, 1996.

Kurchak, Sarah. "I'm Autistic, and Believe Me, It's a Lot Better than Measles." *Archipelago*, February 6, 2015.

L. B. "Nationaltheatret." Program Notes.

Laffan, William M. " 'Miss Mary Shaw in "Ghosts.' " *The Sun*, January 27, 1903.

Latham, Baldwin. *The Utilisation of* Sewage. London: E and F. N., 1867.

Lawlor, Christopher. *Consumption and Literature: The Making of a Romantic Disease*. Basingstoke: Palgrave Macmillan, 2006.

Leavitt, Judith Walzer. *Brought to Bed: Childbearing in America 1750 to 1950*. New York: Oxford University Press, 1986.

Leavy, Barbara Fass. *To Blight with Plague*. New York: New York University Press, 1992.

Lepke, Arno K. "Who is Doctor Stockmann?" *Scandinavian Studies* 32, no. 2 (1960): 59.

Levine, George. *Realism, Ethics, and Secularism: Essays on Victorian Literature and Science*. Cambridge: Cambridge University Press, 2008.

Licencing Prositution. London: Unwin Bros., 1869.

Liggins, Emma. "Writing against the 'Husband-Fiend'; Syphilis and Male Sexual Vice in the New Woman Novel." *Women's Writing* 7, no. 2 (2000): 175–95.

Lindholdt, Paul. "Greening the Dramatic Canon: Henrik Ibsen's 'An Enemy of the People.' " *Interdisciplinary Literary Studies* 3, no. 1 (2001): 56.

McFarlane, James, ed. *The Cambridge Companion to Ibsen.* Cambridge: Cambridge University Press, 1994.

Machiraju, A. F. "Ideals and Victims: Ibsen's Concerns in *Ghosts* and *The Wild Duck.*" *Modern Language Review* 87, no. 1 (1992): 134–42.

McWhir, Anne. "Mary Shelley's Anti-Contagionism: *The Last Man* as 'Fatal Narrative.'" *Mosaic: An Interdisciplinary Critical Journal* 35, no. 2 (2002): 23–38.

Matos, Timothy Carlo. "Choleric Fictions: Epidemiology, Medical Authority, and *An Enemy of the People.*" *Modern Drama* 51, no. 3 (2008): 353–68.

Martin, Emily. *The Woman in the Body: A Cultural Analysis of Reproduction.* Boston: Beacon Press, 2001.

Matz, Aaron. *Satire in an Age of Realism.* Cambridge: Cambridge University Press, 2010.

Meier, Thomas Keith. *Defoe and the Defense of Commerce.* Victoria: University of Victoria Press, 1987.

Melville, Peter. "The Problem of Immunity in *The Last Man.*" *SEL* 47, no. 4 (2007).

Meredith, George. *The Egoist.* New York: Norton, 1979.

———. *The Ordeal of Richard Feverel.*

Michaelson, Karen L. *Childbirth in America: Anthropological Perspectives.* South Hadley: Bergin and Garvey, 1988.

Miller, Arthur. "A Letter from Arthur Miller." *An Enemy of the People* Theater program, February 1971.

Miller, J. Hillis. *The Disappearance of God: Five Nineteenth-Century Writers.* Cambridge: Harvard University Press, 1963.

Miller, William Ian. *The Anatomy of Disgust.* Cambridge: Harvard University Press, 1997.

Miss Mitford. "Female Friendship." *The Literary Panorama,* May 1813.

"More Morbid than Ibsen." *Saturday Review,* February 24, 1894.

Newman, Francis W. *The Cure of the Great Social Evil, with Special Reference to Recent Laws Delusively Called Contagious Diseases' Acts.* London: Trubner, 1869).

"New Theatrical Bills." *New York Times* April 9, 1895.

Nuland, Sherwin B. "The Enigma of Semmelweis—an Interpretation." Commentary in *The Etiology, The Concept, and the Prophylaxis of Childbed Fever.*" Birmingham: Classics of Medicine Library, 1981.

Nylenna, Magne. "Dr. Stockman nog dr. Snow—to samfunnsmedisinske helter." *Tidsskriftet: Den Norske Legeforening,* December 18, 2003.

Oliphant, Margaret. "The Anti-Marriage League." *Blackwood's,* January 1896.

Otis, Laura. *Membranes: Metaphors of Invasion in Nineteenth-Century Literature, Science, and Politics.* Baltimore: Johns Hopkins University Press, 1999.

Ott, Katherine. *Fevered Lives: Tuberculosis in American Culture since 1870.* Boston: Harvard University Press, 199.

"Passages from the Diary of a Late Physician: Consumption." *Museum of Foreign Literature,* January 1831.

Pearson, Karl. *Tuberculosis, Heredity, and Environment.* 1912.

Poore, G. V. *Dry methods of Sanitation.* London: Edward Stanford, 1894.

Postlewait, Thomas. *Prophet of the New Drama: William Archer and the Ibsen Campaign.* Westport: Greenwood, 1985.

Quétel, Claude. *History of Syphilis.* Translated by Judith Braddock and Brian Pike. Cambridge: Polity Press, 1990.

"Recent Fiction." *The Critic,* April 16, 1887.

Redmond, James. *Madness in Drama.* Cambridge: Cambridge University Press, 1993.

The Remedy Worse than the Disease. London: 1869.

Review of "An Enemy of the People." *The Referee,* July 22, 1894.

Richetti, John J. *Daniel Defoe.* Boston: Twayne, 1987.

Rivers, W. C. "Marriage and Tuberculosis." *Saturday Review,* March 15, 1902.

Romano, Terrie M. "The Cattle Plague of 1865 and the Reception of 'The Germ Theory' in Mid-Victorian Britain." *Journal of the History of Medicine* 52 (1997): 51–80.

Rooks, Judith Pence. *Midwifery and Childbirth in America.* Philadelphia: Temple University Press, 1997.

Roosen, William James. *Daniel Defoe and Diplomacy.* Selinsgrove: Susquehanna University Press, 1986.

Rothman, Barbara Katz. *In Labor: Women and Power in the Birthplace.* New York: Norton, 1982.

Russell, William L. "Consumption: The Conditions Which Invite a Foothold of this Dread Disease." *Maine Farmer,* February 4, 1897.

Russett, Cynthia Eagle. *Sexual Science.* Cambridge: Harvard University Press, 1989.

Salomé, Lou. *Ibsen's Heroines.* Edited and translated by Siegfried Mandel. Redding Ridge: Black Swan Books, 1985.

Seager, Nicholas. "Lies, Damned Lies, and Statistics: Epistemology and Fiction in Defoe's *A Journal of the Plague Year.*" *Modern Language Review* 103, no. 3 (2008): 639–53.

Semmelweis, Ignaz. *The Etiology, Concept and Prophylaxis of Childbed Fever.* Translated by K. Codell Carter. Madison: University of Wisconsin Press, 1983.

Schaffer, Talia. *The Forgotten Female Aesthetes: Literary Culture in Late-Victorian England.* Charlottesville: University of Virginia Press, 2000.

Scheiber, Andrew. "The Doctor's Order: Eugenic Anxiety in Henry James's *Washington Square.*" *Literature and Medicine* 15, no. 2 (1996): 244–62.

Schoenfeld, Lois Beth. *Dysfunctional Families in the Wessex Novels of Thomas Hardy.* Lanham: University Press of America, 2005.

Schreiber, Werner. *Infectio: Infectious Diseases in the History of Medicine.* Basle: Hoffman-La Rouche, 1987.

Shaw, George Bernard. *The Doctor's Dilemma.* New York: Penguin, 1957.

———. *Quintessence of Ibsenism.* New York: Hill and Wang, 1958.

Shaw, John. *Antiseptics in Obstetric Nursing.* London: H. K. Lewis, 1890.

Shelley, Mary. *The Last Man*. Hertfordshire: Wordsworth Classics, 2004.

Shelley, Percy. *Adonais*.

Shideler, Ross. *Questioning the Father: From Darwin to Zola, Ibsen, Strindberg, and Hardy*. Stanford: Stanford University Press, 1999.

Shorter, Edward. *A History of Women's Bodies*. New York: Basic Books, 1982.

Shrewsbury, J. F. D. *A History of the Bubonic Plague in the British Isles*. Cambridge: Harvard University Press, 1970.

Shuttleworth, Sally. "The Psychology of Childhood in Victorian Literature and Medicine." In *Literature, Science, Psychoanalysis, 1830–1970*, edited by Gillian Beer, Helen Small, and Trudi Tate, 86–101. Oxford: Oxford University Press, 2003.

"Sierra Leone Loses Its 10th Doctor to Ebola Outbreak." *CBSNews.com*, December 7, 2014.

Smith, Andrew. *Victorian Demons: Medicine, Masculinity, and the Gothic at the fin-de-siècle*. Manchester: Manchester University Press, 2004.

Smith, J. Anderson. "Immunity from Disease." *The Wesleyan-Methodist Magazine*, June 1893.

Sontag, Susan. *Illness as Metaphor*. New York: McGraw-Hill, 1978.

Sparham, Legard. *Reasons against the Practice of Inoculating the Small-Pox*. London: Peele, 1722.

Spencer, Thomas. *On the Quality of the New River Company's Water*. London: Gilbert and Rivington, 1855.

Spongberg, Mary. *Feminizing Venereal Disease: The Body of the Prostitute in Nineteenth-Century Medical Discourse*. New York: New York University Press, 1997.

Sprinchorn, Evert. "Syphilis in Ibsen's *Ghosts*." *Ibsen Studies* 4, no. 2 (2004): 191–204.

Stowe, Harriet Beecher. *Uncle Tom's Cabin*. New York: Norton, 1994.

"Successful disinfectant." *Medical and Other Uses of Carbolic Acid*. Manchester: F. C. Calvert.

Sudan, Rajani. *Fair Exotics: Xenophobic Subjects in English Literature, 1720–1850*. Philadelphia: University of Pennsylvania Press, 2002.

———. *Alchemy and Empire: Abject Materials and the Technologies of Colonialism*. New York: Fordham University Press, 2016.

"Syphilitic Child." Wellcome Images. Taken from Franz Mracek, *Atlas of Syphilis and the Venereal Diseases*. London: Rebman, 1898.

Szreter, Simon. *Health and Wealth: Studies in History and Policy*. Rochester: University of Rochester Press, 2007.

Tansey, E. M. "From Germ Theory to 1945." In *Western Medicine: An Illustrated History*, edited by Irvine Loudon, 102–22. Oxford: Oxford University Press, 1997.

Taylor, Charles Bell. *Observations on the Contagious Disease Acts*. Nottingham: 1869.

Templeton, Joan. "Advocacy and Ambivalence in Ibsen's Drama." *Ibsen Studies* 7, no. 1 (2007): 43–60.

Tennyson, Lord Alfred. "The Lady of Shallot."

———. "Mariana."

"*Tess of the D'Urbervilles.*" *Novel Review*, March 1892.

Theater Season Program. "Nationaltheatrets repertoire 1ste season 1899–1900."

Thomson, John. *Victorian London Street Life in Historic Photographs* New York: Dover, 21.

Tomes, N. J., and J. H. Warner. *Rethinking the Reception of the Germ Theory of Disease.* Special issue, *The Journal of the History of Medicine* 52 (1997).

Trotter, David. *Circulation: Defoe, Dickens, and the Economies of the Novel.* New York: St. Martin's, 1988.

Van Laan, Thomas F. "Generic complexity in Ibsen's 'An Enemy of the People.'" *Comparative Drama* 20, no. 2 (1986): 96.

Vapo-Cresolene Vaporizer, product box.

Vardoulakis, Dimitris. "Spectres of Duty: Silence in Ibsen's *Ghosts.*" *Orbis Litterarum* 64, no. 1 (2009): 50–74.

"Vegetable Villains." *Good Words*, December 1883.

Vinten-Johansen, P. "Dr. Stockmann and Dr. Snow." *Tidsskriftet: Den Norske Legeforening*, August 1, 2004.

Vrettos, Athena. *Somatic Fictions: Imagining Illness in Victorian Culture.* Stanford: Stanford University Press, 1995.

Wagner-Lawlor, Jennifer A. "Performing History, Performing Humanity in Mary Shelley's *The Last Man.*" *Studies in English Literature* (Autumn 2002): 769.

Wagstaffe, W. *A Letter to Dr. Friend Shewing the Danger and Uncertainity of Inoculating the Small Pox.* London: Butler, 1722.

Wald, Priscilla. *Contagious: Cultures, Carriers, and the Outbreak Narrative.* Durham: Duke University Press, 2008.

Walkowitz, Judith R. *Prostitution and Victorian Society: Women, Class, and the State.* Cambridge: Cambridge University Press, 1980.

Wall, Cynthia. "Novel Streets: The Rebuilding of London and Defoe's *A Journal of the Plague Year.*" *Studies in the Novel* 30, no. 2 (1998): 164–77.

Wallace, Stephen. "Governing Humanity." *Journal for Medical Humanities* 29 (2008): 29–31.

W. C. "The Germ Theory." *Chambers's Journal of Popular Literature, Science, and Art*, March 4, 1876.

Wellcome Images. Taken from Franz Mracek, *Atlas of Syphilis and the Venereal Diseases.* London: Rebman, 1898.

Wertz, Richard W., and Dorothy C. Wertz. *Lying-In: A History of Childbirth in America.* Expanded ed. New Haven: Yale University Press, 1989.

W. H. P. "The Ibsen Bacillus." *The National Observer*, November 28, 1896.

Wolff, Tamsen. *Mendel's Theatre: Heredity, Eugenics, and Early Twentieth Century American Drama.* Basingstoke: Palgrave, 2009.

"Women's Friendships." *Saturday Review of Politics, Literature, Science and Art*, April, 28, 1866.

Wood, Ellen. *East Lynne.* Oxford: Oxford University Press, 2008.

Woodville, William. *Reports of a Series of Inoculations for the Variolæ Vaccine or Cow-pox.* London: James Phillips and Son, 1799.

Wright, Sarah Bird. *Thomas Hardy A to Z.* New York: Checkmark Books, 2002.

Ystad, Vigdis. *Ibsen at the Centre for Advanced Study.* Oslo: Scandinavian University Press, 1997.

Zimmerman, Barry E., and David J. Zimmerman. *Killer Germs: Microbes and Diseases that Threaten Humanity.* New York: McGraw-Hill, 2003.

Zimmerman, Virginia. *Excavating Victorians.* Albany: State University of New York Press, 2008.

Zwart, Hub. "Environmental Pollution and Professional Responsibility: Ibsen's *A Public Enemy* as a Seminar on Science Communication and Ethics." *Environmental Values* 13 (2004): 364.

Index

www.ingramcontent.com/pod-product-compliance
Lightning Source LLC
Chambersburg PA
CBHW020650030726
47498CB00002B/449